MW00878143

The

DASH DIET

COOKBOOK

FOR BEGINNERS

Unlock the Power of DASH: Simple Steps to Heart Health and Weight Control - Includes a 56-Day Meal Plan, Delicious Recipes, and Weekly Shopping Lists

Ava Fit

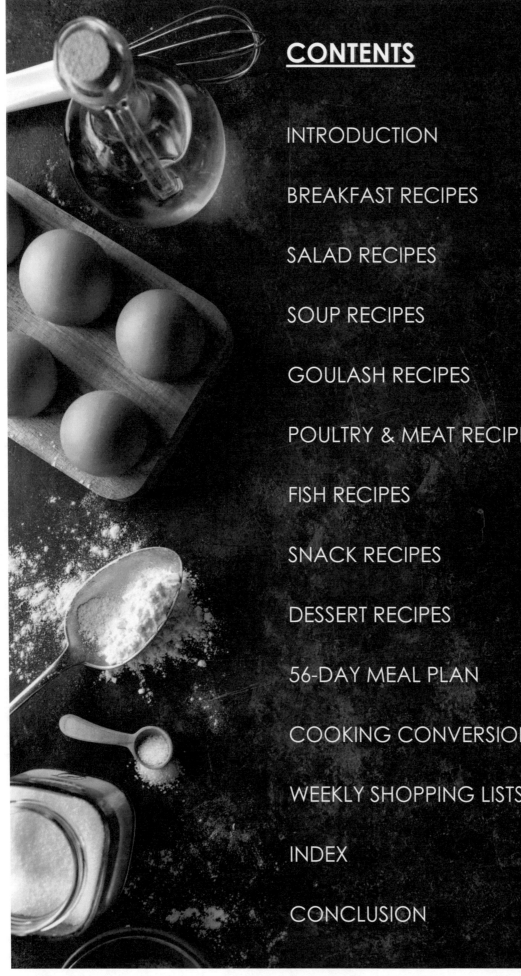

CONTENTS

Introduction

In our bustling modern lives, where days are dominated by screens, deadlines, and the never-ending to-do lists, we often forget the simple joys. Among those joys is the act of indulging in nourishing and flavorful meals. But in the maze of trendy diets and ever-changing health advice, how do we choose the right path? Enter the DASH diet, your trustworthy guide to a healthier life and a steadfast ally against high blood pressure.

Nestled in the heart of health-conscious dietary recommendations, the DASH diet isn't a fleeting trend. It's a carefully researched and well-established eating plan, originally designed to combat hypertension. But as thousands have discovered, its benefits extend far beyond just managing blood pressure levels.

Step into a day in the life of someone on the DASH diet, and you'll see tables laden with vibrant fruits and vegetables, hearty portions of whole grains, lean proteins sourced from both land and sea, and a limited but purposeful use of salt. It's a tableau of food that not only tantalizes the taste buds but also promises a plethora of health benefits.

Diving deeper into what DASH really stands for - Dietary Approaches to Stop Hypertension - it's evident that this isn't just about food. It's a holistic approach to health. And while the name might make it sound technical, at its heart, the DASH diet is straightforward and user-friendly.

The beauty of the DASH diet is its flexibility and adaptability. Whether you're a seasoned chef or someone who struggles to boil an egg, this diet accommodates everyone. You don't need to overhaul your pantry overnight; it's about making gradual changes, understanding the importance of each food group, and finding out how they fit into your unique lifestyle.

With each passing day on the DASH diet, envision your body thanking you. Feel the surge of more energy, the comfort of stable blood pressure readings, and the undeniable glow of good health. This isn't just about numbers on a scale or fleeting compliments. It's about a sustained, long-term commitment to your well-being.

But it's essential to remember that at the core of the DASH diet is the promise of enjoyment. Yes, it's about health, but it's also about relishing the diverse flavors, textures, and experiences that food offers. It's a celebration of meals, an embrace of nutrition, and an invitation to a healthier, happier you.

So, as you turn the pages of this book, get ready to embark on a transformative journey. One where you'll discover not just recipes but a new way of looking at food and health. Welcome to the world of the DASH diet. Your pathway to a vibrant, more fulfilled life starts here.

Understanding High Blood Pressure

In the vast landscape of human health, blood pressure stands as a sentinel, a quiet guardian that holds profound insights into our well-being. Often dubbed the 'silent killer', high blood pressure or hypertension, as it is formally known, is deceptively stealthy. Many traverse through life unaware of its lurking presence, only to face its daunting consequences later on. But by arming ourselves with knowledge and understanding, we can better navigate this challenge.

So, what exactly is blood pressure? Imagine your arteries as garden hoses. When water flows through them at a forceful rate, they feel the pressure. Similarly, when blood courses through your arteries, it exerts pressure on the walls of those vessels. This pressure, essential for blood to deliver oxygen and nutrients to our body, is what we commonly refer to as blood pressure.

However, when this force becomes too strong, persistently, it begins to cause health issues. This heightened state is hypertension. Think of it as a garden hose being constantly filled to its brim, the pressure straining its boundaries. Over time, this continuous strain can lead to severe health complications like heart disease, stroke, and kidney issues.

But how do you know if your blood pressure is high? The tricky part is that hypertension rarely shows clear symptoms. It's not like a cold, where you can feel its effects or see its signs. This is why regular check-ups and monitoring are crucial. It's about listening to the whispers of your body before they become alarming shouts.

The good news is, understanding your blood pressure readings isn't as daunting as it may seem. When you check your blood pressure, you'll get two readings: systolic and diastolic. The systolic number (the higher one) indicates the pressure in your arteries when your heart beats. The diastolic number (the lower one) showcases the pressure when your heart is resting between beats. Both numbers are crucial for assessing your overall blood pressure health.

Now, you might wonder, "What causes high blood pressure?" Several factors play into this. Some are out of our control, like genetics or age. However, many contributors, like diet, activity levels, stress, and lifestyle choices, can be managed. This is where the DASH diet shines as a beacon of hope, offering dietary and lifestyle strategies to combat and control hypertension.

As we delve deeper into this book, we'll not only explore the intricacies of high blood pressure but also arm you with tools, tips, and dietary guidelines to help you lead a balanced, healthier life. Remember, knowledge is the first step towards empowerment. And in understanding high blood pressure, you're taking a pivotal step towards a brighter, healthier future.

Causes of High Blood Pressure

The symphony of our body is a remarkable one, with each part playing its vital role. However, like any intricate system, disruptions can emerge, and in the realm of our health, high blood pressure is a significant concern. To combat it effectively, we must first unravel its root causes. Let's embark on this journey of understanding together.

Genetics and Family History: Sometimes, our genes are the silent scriptwriters of our health story. If your parents or close family members have a history of hypertension, there's a likelihood you might inherit the same predisposition. It's nature's way, but being forewarned means you can be forearmed with proactive measures.

Age: As the pages of our life's book turn, our blood vessels undergo changes. They may stiffen or narrow, leading to increased pressure as blood flows. This natural aging process can elevate the risk of hypertension, especially as we cross significant milestones in our life.

Diet and Sodium Intake: The modern American plate, often laden with processed foods, can be a minefield of excessive sodium. This salt abundance can cause our body to retain water, increasing the volume of blood and, consequently, the pressure.

Lack of Physical Activity: A sedentary lifestyle is akin to an unattended garden. Without regular movement, our heart muscles weaken, compelling it to work harder to pump blood, thus increasing pressure in the arteries.

Excess Weight: Carrying extra pounds, especially around the waist, can strain our heart and blood vessels. This additional burden can lead to a higher blood pressure, making weight management a pivotal aspect of controlling hypertension.

Alcohol and Tobacco Use: Both alcohol and tobacco contain substances that can narrow and make our blood vessels more rigid. Consistent or excessive consumption of either can elevate the risk of high blood pressure, aside from posing other health hazards.

Stress: Our fast-paced lives often come with their set of challenges, leading to chronic stress. This relentless pressure can release stress hormones that temporarily narrow our arteries, causing spikes in blood pressure.

Other Health Conditions: Diseases such as kidney disease, diabetes, and sleep apnea can interfere with our body's mechanisms that regulate blood pressure. Medications, too, like certain pain killers, decongestants, and even birth control pills, can influence our blood pressure levels.

Hormonal Imbalances: Conditions like thyroid problems or adrenal gland tumors can disrupt our body's hormonal balance, which plays a vital role in regulating blood pressure.

Diving into these causes offers us a clear roadmap of potential triggers and influences on our blood pressure. However, with this knowledge in hand, the power to change, adapt, and embrace healthier choices becomes attainable. As we navigate through the subsequent chapters, we'll discover how the DASH diet can act as a guiding light, leading us away from these pitfalls and towards a future of health and vitality.

What is the DASH Diet?

In a world where fad diets emerge as quickly as they fade, the DASH diet stands out not just as another trend but as a medically endorsed approach to healthier living. The name 'DASH' is an acronym for *Dietary Approaches to Stop Hypertension*. As the name suggests, its primary purpose was to combat high blood pressure, but the numerous health benefits it offers extend far beyond that.

Originating from research funded by the U.S. National Institutes of Health, the DASH diet has been meticulously crafted based on scientific evidence. It's not just another diet – it's a lifelong commitment to a healthier you.

Unlike many restrictive diets, DASH doesn't ask you to give up on entire food groups or live on juice cleanses. Instead, it emphasizes a balanced consumption of the right foods in the right proportions. Picture this: plates filled with colorful vegetables, whole grains, lean protein, and a dash of dairy. Fresh fruits as snacks, and nuts and legumes sprinkled into your routine. It's not about deprivation, but moderation and making smart choices.

Central to the DASH philosophy is the reduction of sodium intake. The average American diet is saturated with salt, far exceeding the recommended daily limit. By moderating salt and increasing the intake of foods rich in magnesium, potassium, and calcium, DASH aims to regulate blood pressure and fortify overall health.

An added bonus? Weight management becomes a natural byproduct. As you immerse yourself in the wholesome goodness of nutrient-dense foods, empty calories and junk foods lose their allure. With DASH, you don't just lose weight, you nurture a healthier relationship with food.

The beauty of the DASH diet is its adaptability. Whether you're a young athlete, a busy parent, or navigating the golden years, DASH offers a roadmap to a more nutritious lifestyle, tailored to individual needs. By focusing on fresh, natural ingredients and mindful eating, DASH isn't just a diet—it's a movement towards holistic well-being.

Joining the DASH journey doesn't mean a drastic overhaul of your kitchen or habits overnight. It's about gradual change, making one smart choice at a time, and appreciating the joy of nourishing meals. The goal isn't merely to live longer but to live better, with vitality and zest. And with the DASH diet, this vision is entirely achievable.

How the DASH Diet Helps Control Blood Pressure

Understanding our blood pressure is pivotal to grasping our heart's well-being. When our readings edge upwards, it's an alarming whisper of underlying concerns, even if we feel perfectly fine on the outside. These elevated levels, if unchecked, can pave the way to grave heart-related complications. Enter the DASH diet – a strategic, science-backed approach specifically designed to rein in these escalating numbers and ensure our heart beats with vitality and vigor.

Lower Sodium Intake: Sodium is a common culprit in the hypertension story. The typical American diet often involves high sodium intake, primarily due to processed foods and excessive seasoning. DASH puts a firm foot down on high salt content. By encouraging fresh, unprocessed foods and offering flavorful alternatives to salt, this diet ensures your sodium levels stay in check, naturally aiding in blood pressure regulation.

Rich in Potassium, Magnesium, and Calcium: These three essential minerals play a crucial role in blood pressure control. The DASH diet promotes foods like bananas, beans, nuts, leafy greens, and dairy – all of which are powerhouses of these minerals. Regular consumption can help balance the body's sodium-potassium ratio, assisting in the relaxation and contraction of blood vessels, which in turn stabilizes blood pressure.

High Fiber Content: Fiber is often celebrated for its digestive benefits, but it's equally crucial for heart health. The DASH diet is teeming with whole grains, fruits, and vegetables, ensuring a healthy dose of fiber in every meal. Fiber aids in maintaining a healthy weight and reduces harmful cholesterol levels, both of which are key players in blood pressure management.

Lean Proteins: Ditching fatty cuts of meat for leaner options like poultry, fish, beans, and tofu can make a significant difference. These sources not only provide essential proteins for body repair and growth but also contain fewer saturated fats, helping keep your arteries clear and flexible, facilitating smoother blood flow and healthier pressure levels.

Healthy Fats: All fats aren't bad. The DASH diet champions the consumption of beneficial fats found in avocados, nuts, seeds, and olive oil. These fats can help reduce the "bad" LDL cholesterol, making way for improved arterial health, and consequently, more stabilized blood pressure readings.

Limiting Alcohol and Caffeine: Both can be enjoyed in moderation, but excessive intake can spike blood pressure levels. The DASH approach recommends judicious consumption, balancing pleasure with health priorities.

Promotion of a Holistic Lifestyle: Beyond the plate, DASH also promotes a balanced lifestyle. Stress is a silent trigger for hypertension. By advocating for regular physical activity, adequate rest, and mindfulness practices, the DASH approach ensures the body and mind work harmoniously, resulting in optimal blood pressure levels.

In essence, the DASH diet is more than a mere dietary plan. It's a comprehensive lifestyle transformation with the singular goal of nurturing cardiovascular health. When one adopts the principles of DASH, they're not just embracing a diet; they're making a commitment to a heart-happier, pressure-balanced life.

Products and Recommendations for the DASH Diet

When embarking on the DASH journey, it's imperative to have a clear road map – knowing which foods to embrace and which ones to limit or avoid. It's not about deprivation but making smarter, heart-friendly choices that can become a natural part of your daily routine. So, let's delve into the core components of the DASH diet and understand the guidelines that make it so effective.

1. Whole Grains: Whole grains are the foundation of the DASH diet. Instead of refined grains that have been stripped of their natural nutrients, whole grains retain their fibrous bran, nutritious germ, and starchy endosperm. Examples include brown rice, quinoa, barley, and whole wheat bread. These grains provide sustained energy and are packed with fiber, which aids digestion and keeps you feeling full.

2. Vegetables: The DASH diet emphasizes a bounty of colorful and nutrient-rich vegetables. From leafy greens to crunchy bell peppers, the more variety, the better. These foods are abundant in essential vitamins, minerals, and antioxidants that bolster our health.

3. Fruits: Much like vegetables, fruits are a cornerstone of the DASH diet. They offer a sweet alternative to processed sugary treats and are loaded with beneficial compounds, vitamins, and fibers. Whether it's the potassium in bananas or the vitamin C in oranges, fruits play a pivotal role in balancing our blood pressure.

4. Dairy: When it comes to dairy on the DASH diet, think low-fat or non-fat options. These provide the calcium and protein we need without the added saturated fats. Yogurts, milk, and cheese are all on the menu, just in their leaner versions.

5. Lean Meats, Poultry, and Fish: Protein is an essential building block for our bodies, and the DASH diet recommends lean sources. Think of fish like salmon, which is rich in omega-3 fatty acids, or skinless chicken breasts. Red meats are not off-limits but should be consumed in moderation.

6. Nuts, Seeds, and Legumes: These are not only excellent protein sources but also packed with vital nutrients and healthy fats. Whether it's the magnesium in almonds, the fiber in lentils, or the healthy fats in walnuts, incorporating these into your diet can offer multiple health benefits.

7. Fats and Oils: Healthy fats are encouraged in the DASH diet. Olive oil, avocados, and nuts contain monounsaturated and polyunsaturated fats, which can help reduce bad cholesterol levels. However, it's essential to moderate intake, ensuring that fats make up only about 27% of your daily caloric intake.

8. Sweets: The DASH diet doesn't deprive you of life's sweet pleasures but advises moderation. When indulging, choose treats that are low in added sugars and fats. It's all about balance and making informed decisions.

9. Sodium: One of the most critical aspects of the DASH diet is reducing sodium intake. Too much salt can lead to water retention and increased blood pressure. The recommendation is to limit sodium to 2,300 mg a day or ideally, if you can, aim for a stricter 1,500 mg.

In essence, the DASH diet is about harmony and balance. It's a guide to infusing our daily intake with nutrient-rich, wholesome foods that not only cater to our palate but also nurture our heart and overall health. With these guidelines in hand, you're equipped to make choices that can profoundly impact your well-being.

Tips and Tricks

Welcome to the heart of the DASH diet — a place where I want you to feel equipped, inspired, and ready to make every meal a step toward better health. Here, I've compiled essential tidbits to help you maximize the benefits of this dietary approach and navigate any challenges that might come your way.

1. Embracing the DASH Tips

The beauty of the DASH diet lies not only in its proven health benefits but also in its flexibility. While the recipes provided in this book are tailored to meet DASH guidelines, I encourage you to see them as starting points. Feel free to tweak them to cater to your palate or to make use of the fresh produce available in your region. Remember:

- Every individual's nutritional needs can vary. Listen to your body and consult with a healthcare professional if you have specific dietary concerns.
- Track your progress. Sometimes, it's the small victories — like reducing your salt intake gradually — that lead to lasting change.
- Stay hydrated. Along with monitoring your salt and nutrient intake, drinking ample water is pivotal in maintaining balanced blood pressure levels.

2. Navigating Salt and Its Substitutes

We often hear "salt to taste" in culinary circles, but the DASH diet encourages mindfulness about sodium intake. Here's what you need to know:

Exact Sodium Counts: Instead of leaving it to guesswork, I've mentioned precise sodium amounts in our recipes. This helps ensure you're within the DASH-recommended limits.

Salt Substitutes: If you're aiming to further reduce your salt consumption, consider herbs like rosemary, thyme, or oregano, and spices like cumin, paprika, or garlic powder to amplify flavors. Lemon juice or vinegar can also give a dish that extra zing without the sodium punch. Remember, it's about balancing flavor without compromising health.

3. Incorporating Additional Ingredients

The beauty of cooking lies in experimentation. While my recipes provide a robust DASH-friendly foundation, there's always room for creativity:

- **Seasonal Produce**: Consider adding vegetables or fruits that are in season. They're not only fresher but often more flavorful and nutrient-rich.
- **Pairings**: Think about texture and taste. A crunchy nut might complement a creamy dish, or a tangy fruit could elevate a savory plate.
- **Nutritional Boosts**: Ingredients like flaxseeds, chia seeds, or unsweetened cocoa can add a healthful punch without straying from DASH guidelines. Do keep an eye on portion sizes, though!

4. Equip Yourself for Success

Cooking is more than just following a recipe; it's an experience. Invest in quality kitchen tools and appliances that make the process enjoyable. A good knife, efficient blender, or a reliable pressure cooker can be game-changers in your DASH journey.

Lastly, surround yourself with a support system — be it family, friends, or online communities. Share your successes, seek advice during challenges, and remember, every meal is a step toward a healthier you.

How to Use This Book

Navigating through a cookbook, especially one focused on a particular diet, can be a journey of its own. Here's a brief guide to ensure you effortlessly sail through these pages and make the most of every recipe and tip I've provided:

1. Recipes: Each recipe in this book offers you a snapshot of the time you'll spend: preparation time, cooking time, and the total time required. For dishes that demand additional time — like marination or waiting periods — you'll find these durations explicitly mentioned. Accompanying every recipe is a vibrant photo that provides a visual representation of the final dish, a detailed list of ingredients, and step-by-step cooking instructions. Additionally, each recipe features a 'Nutrition' and 'Equipment' section to provide clarity on nutritional content and the tools you'll need.

2. Meal Plan: The heart of the DASH journey lies in the meals you consume. The meal plan comprises titles for breakfasts, lunches, dinners, desserts, and snacks. For ease of reference, I've tagged each recipe title with its corresponding page number. An exclusive column within the meal plan also provides the calorie count for each daily meal, ensuring you stay within your nutritional goals.

3. Weekly Shopping Lists: Staying organized is the key to sticking to any diet. Each weekly shopping list encompasses a detailed inventory of ingredients, along with their required quantities, mapped to the meals in the corresponding week's meal plan. This ensures that your grocery trips are efficient and that you have everything on hand when it's time to cook.

4. Glossary: For quick navigation, the glossary lists all the recipes alphabetically with their respective page numbers. Whether you're looking for a familiar favorite or wanting to try something new, the glossary will point you in the right direction.

5. Cooking Conversion Chart: Because measurements matter in cooking, this section comprises tables for:

- Dry Volume Equivalents
- Liquid Volume Equivalents
- Temperature Equivalents
- Weight Equivalents

It ensures that your measurements are precise, aiding in the successful execution of each recipe.

In closing, I hope this book becomes your trusty companion in the kitchen, guiding you towards healthier eating habits and a vibrant lifestyle. Enjoy every bite, cherish every moment, and remember — good health is the ultimate recipe for happiness.

Bon Appétit!

Honey Drizzle Oatmeal with Fresh Berries

Prep time: 5 min   **Total time:** 15 min
Cook time: 10 min   **Servings:** 2

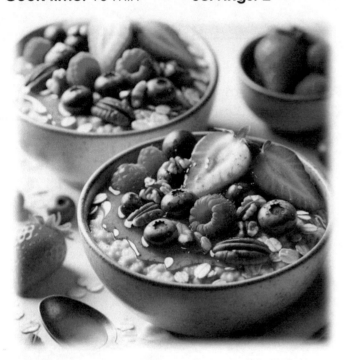

Ingredients:

✓ Rolled oats: 1 cup
✓ Water: 2 cups
✓ Salt: pinch
✓ Honey: 2 tbsp
✓ Mixed fresh berries (strawberries, blueberries, raspberries): 1/2 cup
✓ Chopped nuts (almonds, walnuts, or pecans): 1/4 cup

Directions:

1. In a saucepan, bring water to a boil. Add a pinch of salt.
2. Stir in the rolled oats. Reduce heat and simmer, stirring occasionally, until oats are soft and have absorbed the water, about 5-7 minutes.
3. Divide the oatmeal into two bowls.

4. Drizzle each bowl with 1 tablespoon of honey.
5. Top with fresh berries and chopped nuts.
6. Serve immediately and enjoy!

Nutrition: Calories: 220; Fat: 6g; Carbs: 38g; Protein: 7g; Sugar: 14g; Fiber: 5g;

Equipment: Saucepan; Stirring spoon; Bowls; Measuring cups and spoons.

Mango Greek Yogurt with Toasted Walnuts

Prep time: 10 min   **Total time:** 15 min
Cook time: 5 min   **Servings:** 2

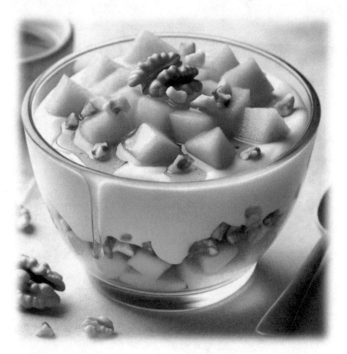

Ingredients:

✓ Greek yogurt: 2 cups
✓ Fresh mango: 1, diced
✓ Honey: 2 tbsp
✓ Toasted walnuts: 1/4 cup

Directions:

1. Start by toasting the walnuts in a dry skillet over medium heat. Stir frequently to avoid burning. This should take about 3-5 minutes.
2. In a serving bowl, layer Greek yogurt at the bottom.

3. Add diced mango on top.
4. Drizzle honey over the mango.
5. Finish off with a sprinkle of toasted walnuts.
6. Serve immediately and enjoy!

Nutrition: Calories: 300; Fat: 12g; Carbs: 36g; Protein: 15g; Sugar: 28g; Fiber: 3g;

Equipment: Skillet; Serving bowl; Spoon; Knife; Cutting board;

3. Arrange the sliced fresh figs on top of the cottage cheese.
4. Drizzle honey over the figs.
5. Garnish with mint leaves if desired.
6. Serve immediately and enjoy!

Nutrition: Calories: 250; Fat: 5g; Carbs: 40g; Protein: 12g; Sugar: 20g; Fiber: 5g;

Equipment: Toaster; Knife; Spoon; Serving plate.

Fresh Fig and Cottage Cheese Toast

Prep time: 5 min
Cook time: 2 min
Total time: 7 min
Servings: 2

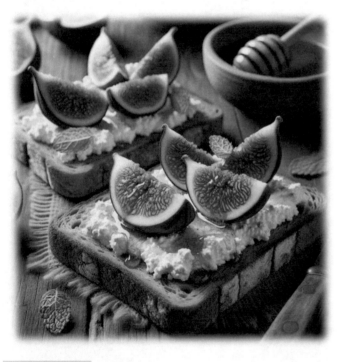

Ingredients:

✓ Whole grain bread: 2 slices
✓ Cottage cheese: 1 cup
✓ Fresh figs: 4, sliced
✓ Honey: 2 tbsp
✓ Mint leaves (optional): a few for garnish

Directions:

1. Toast the whole grain bread slices until they are golden and crispy.
2. Spread a generous layer of cottage cheese on each toast slice.

Broccoli and Mozzarella Omelette

Prep time: 10 min
Cook time: 10 min
Total time: 20 min
Servings: 2

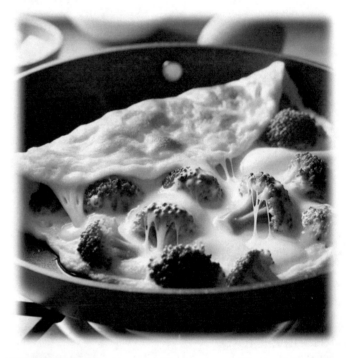

Ingredients:

✓ Eggs, 4
✓ Broccoli, 1 cup (chopped)
✓ Mozzarella cheese, 1/2 cup (shredded)
✓ Salt, to taste
✓ Black pepper, to taste
✓ Olive oil, 1 tbsp

Directions:

1. In a bowl, whisk the eggs, salt, and black pepper until well combined.

2. In a non-stick skillet, heat the olive oil over medium heat. Add the chopped broccoli and sauté until it turns vibrant green and slightly tender.
3. Pour the egg mixture over the broccoli in the skillet. Cook for about 4-5 minutes, until the edges start to lift.
4. Sprinkle the shredded mozzarella cheese evenly over the half side of the omelette.
5. Carefully fold the omelette in half, covering the cheese. Cook for another 2-3 minutes, until the cheese is melted and the omelette is golden brown.
6. Slide the omelette onto a plate, cut in half, and serve immediately.

Nutrition: Calories: 280; Fat: 18g; Carbs: 6g; Protein: 23g; Sugar: 2g; Fiber: 2g;

Equipment: Non-stick skillet; Mixing bowl; Whisk; Spatula.

Apple and Cinnamon Whole Wheat Pita Pockets

Prep time: 15 min **Total time:** 15 min
Cook time: 0 min **Servings:** 4

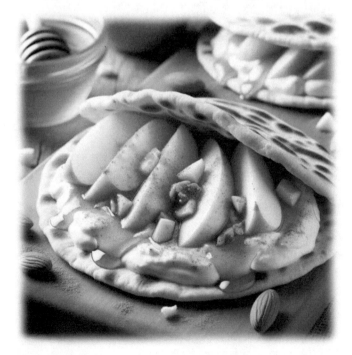

Ingredients:

✓ Whole wheat pita pockets, 4

✓ Fresh apples, 2 (cored and thinly sliced)
✓ Greek yogurt, 1 cup
✓ Honey, 2 tbsp
✓ Cinnamon, 1 tsp
✓ Chopped nuts (e.g. walnuts or almonds), 1/2 cup

Directions:

1. In a small mixing bowl, combine Greek yogurt, honey, and cinnamon. Mix until well combined.
2. Gently open the pita pockets.
3. Spread the yogurt mixture inside each pocket.
4. Insert the sliced apples into the pockets.
5. Sprinkle with chopped nuts.
6. Serve immediately and enjoy!

Nutrition: Calories: 230; Fat: 4g; Carbs: 42g; Protein: 8g; Sugar: 20g; Fiber: 6g;

Equipment: Small mixing bowl; Knife; Spoon.

Barley Breakfast Bowl with Pumpkin Seeds

Prep time: 10 min **Total time:** 40 min
Cook time: 30 min **Servings:** 4

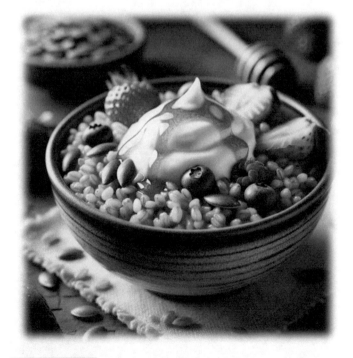

Ingredients:

- ✓ Barley, 1 cup
- ✓ Water, 2 cups
- ✓ Salt, 1 pinch
- ✓ Honey, 2 tbsp
- ✓ Greek yogurt, 1 cup
- ✓ Pumpkin seeds, 1/2 cup
- ✓ Mixed fresh berries, 1 cup

Directions:

1. In a medium-sized saucepan, bring the water to a boil. Add barley and salt.
2. Reduce heat to low, cover, and simmer for approximately 30 minutes or until the barley is tender.
3. Once cooked, remove from heat and let it cool for a few minutes.
4. Transfer the barley to serving bowls.
5. Top with Greek yogurt, honey, pumpkin seeds, and mixed fresh berries.
6. Serve immediately.

Nutrition: Calories: 280; Fat: 6g; Carbs: 48g; Protein: 9g; Sugar: 15g; Fiber: 8g;

Equipment: Medium-sized saucepan; Spoon; Serving bowls.

Baked Beans on Whole Grain Toast

Prep time: 5 min
Cook time: 10 min
Total time: 15 min
Servings: 2

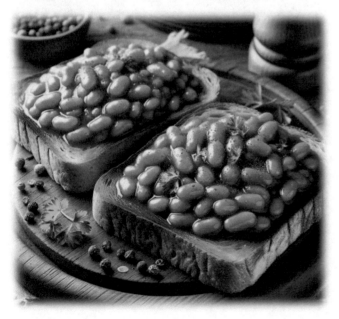

Ingredients:

- ✓ Canned baked beans, 1 cup
- ✓ Whole grain bread, 2 slices
- ✓ Olive oil, 1 tbsp
- ✓ Salt, a pinch
- ✓ Black pepper, to taste
- ✓ Chopped fresh parsley (for garnish), 1 tbsp

Directions:

1. Preheat a skillet over medium heat and add the olive oil.
2. Pour the canned baked beans into the skillet, season with salt and black pepper. Allow to simmer for about 5-7 minutes, stirring occasionally.
3. While the beans are simmering, toast the whole grain bread slices to your desired crispiness.
4. Once toasted, place the slices on a plate.
5. Pour the simmered baked beans over the toast.
6. Garnish with chopped fresh parsley.
7. Serve immediately and enjoy!

Nutrition: Calories: 280; Fat: 7g; Carbs: 44g; Protein: 11g; Sugar: 5g; Fiber: 8g;

Equipment: Skillet; Toaster or Oven; Spoon; Serving plate.

Zucchini and Cottage Cheese Pancakes

Prep time: 15 min
Cook time: 20 min
Total time: 35 min
Servings: 4

Ingredients:

- ✓ Zucchini, grated, 2 cups
- ✓ Cottage cheese, 1 cup
- ✓ Eggs, 2
- ✓ Olive oil, 2 tbsp
- ✓ Salt, a pinch
- ✓ Black pepper, to taste
- ✓ All-purpose flour, 1/2 cup
- ✓ Baking powder, 1 tsp

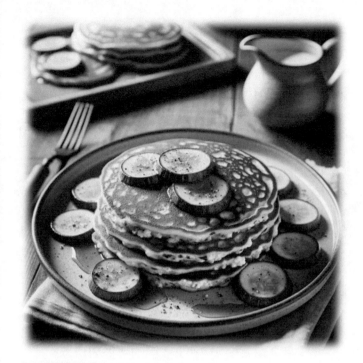

Directions:

1. In a large bowl, combine the grated zucchini, cottage cheese, and eggs. Mix until well combined.
2. Add in the all-purpose flour, baking powder, salt, and black pepper. Stir until the mixture forms a batter.
3. Preheat a skillet over medium heat and add a tablespoon of olive oil.
4. Once the oil is hot, scoop out portions of the batter and drop them into the skillet.
5. Flatten the scoops slightly to form pancakes.
6. Cook each side for about 3-4 minutes or until golden brown.
7. Transfer the cooked pancakes to a plate and repeat with the remaining batter.
8. Serve warm with a dollop of Greek yogurt or a drizzle of honey, if desired.

Nutrition: Calories: 210; Fat: 9g; Carbs: 20g; Protein: 11g; Sugar: 4g; Fiber: 1g;

Equipment: Large mixing bowl; Grater; Skillet; Spatula.

Baked Portobello Mushrooms with Eggs and Herbs

Prep time: 10 min   **Total time:** 25 min
Cook time: 15 min   **Servings:** 4

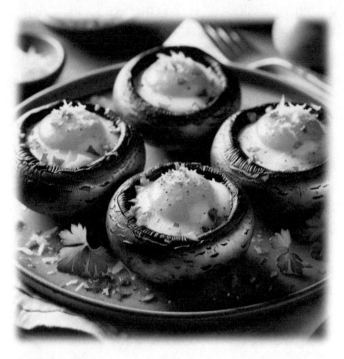

Ingredients:

✓ Portobello mushrooms, 4 large caps
✓ Eggs, 4
✓ Olive oil, 2 tbsp
✓ Chopped fresh parsley, 2 tbsp
✓ Salt, a pinch
✓ Black pepper, to taste
✓ Grated Parmesan cheese (optional), 1/4 cup

Directions:

1. Preheat your oven to 375°F (190°C).
2. Clean the Portobello mushrooms by wiping them with a damp cloth and remove the stems.
3. Drizzle olive oil over the mushroom caps and season with salt and pepper.
4. Place the mushrooms cap-side down on a baking tray.
5. Carefully break an egg into each mushroom cap.
6. Sprinkle chopped parsley and Parmesan cheese (if using) over the eggs.

7. Bake in the preheated oven for 12-15 minutes or until the egg whites are set but the yolks remain runny.
8. Remove from oven and let cool for a minute. Serve hot.

Nutrition: Calories: 180; Fat: 12g; Carbs: 4g; Protein: 11g; Sugar: 1g; Fiber: 1g;

Equipment: Baking tray; Oven; Brush or cloth for cleaning mushrooms.

Spinach and Tomato Breakfast Wraps

Prep time: 10 min
Cook time: 5 min

Total time: 15 min
Servings: 4

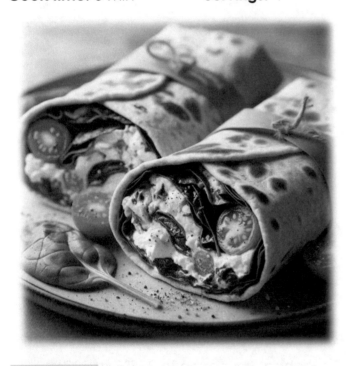

Ingredients:

✓ Whole wheat pita pockets, 4 pcs
✓ Fresh spinach, 2 cups
✓ Cherry tomatoes, 1 cup (halved)
✓ Eggs, 4 pcs
✓ Olive oil, 2 tbsp
✓ Salt, a pinch
✓ Black pepper, to taste
✓ Grated Parmesan cheese, 1/2 cup
✓ Greek yogurt, 1/2 cup (optional for serving)

Directions:

1. Heat the olive oil in a large skillet over medium heat.
2. Add the fresh spinach and cook until wilted, about 2-3 minutes.
3. Push the spinach to one side of the skillet and add the halved cherry tomatoes, cooking for another 2 minutes.
4. In a bowl, whisk the eggs with salt and black pepper.
5. Pour the beaten eggs into the skillet and scramble with the spinach and tomatoes until just set.
6. Warm the pita pockets in the oven or microwave for about 20 seconds.
7. Stuff each pita pocket with the egg, spinach, and tomato mixture.
8. Sprinkle some grated Parmesan cheese inside each wrap.
9. Serve hot with a side of Greek yogurt if desired.

Nutrition: Calories: 295; Fat: 15g; Carbs: 25g; Protein: 15g; Sugar: 3g; Fiber: 4g;

Equipment: Large skillet; Bowl; Whisk; Oven or microwave.

Multi-seed Whole Grain Scones with Fresh Fruit

Prep time: 20 min
Cook time: 25 min

Total time: 45 min
Servings: 8

Ingredients:

✓ All-purpose flour, 1 cup
✓ Rolled oats, 1 cup
✓ Baking powder, 2 tsp
✓ Salt, 1 pinch
✓ Cinnamon, 1/2 tsp
✓ Honey, 3 tbsp
✓ Olive oil, 4 tbsp
✓ Eggs, 2 pcs
✓ Mixed fresh berries (like blueberries, strawberries, raspberries), 1 cup
✓ Pumpkin seeds, 1/4 cup

- ✓ Chopped nuts (like almonds, walnuts), ½ cup
- ✓ Water, 2 tbsp (or as needed)

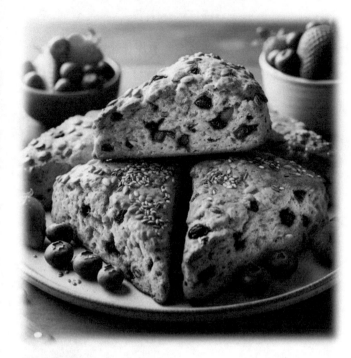

Directions:

1. Preheat your oven to 375°F (190°C) and line a baking sheet with parchment paper.
2. In a large bowl, mix together the all-purpose flour, rolled oats, baking powder, salt, and cinnamon.
3. In another bowl, whisk together honey, olive oil, and eggs.
4. Slowly add the wet mixture into the dry ingredients and mix until just combined.
5. Fold in the mixed fresh berries, pumpkin seeds, and chopped nuts.
6. If the dough is too dry, add water, one tablespoon at a time, until it comes together.
7. Turn the dough out onto a lightly floured surface and shape into an 8-inch round.
8. Cut into 8 wedges and transfer to the prepared baking sheet.
9. Bake for 20-25 minutes or until golden brown.
10. Serve warm with additional fresh berries on top.

Nutrition: Calories: 280; Fat: 12g; Carbs: 35g; Protein: 7g; Sugar: 10g; Fiber: 4g;

Equipment: Baking sheet; Parchment paper; Two large mixing bowls; Whisk; Knife.

Raspberry and Oat Smoothie

Prep time: 5 min   **Total time:** 5 min
Cook time: 0 min   **Servings:** 2

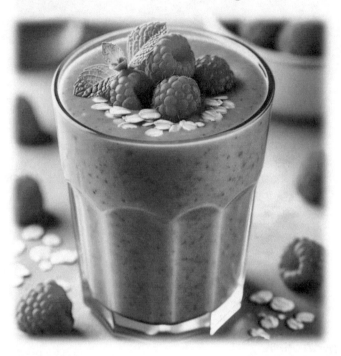

Ingredients:

- ✓ Fresh raspberries, 1 cup
- ✓ Rolled oats, 1/2 cup
- ✓ Greek yogurt, 1 cup
- ✓ Honey, 2 tbsp
- ✓ Water, 1/2 cup
- ✓ Mint leaves, 4 leaves (optional for garnish)

Directions:

1. In a blender, combine fresh raspberries, rolled oats, Greek yogurt, honey, and water.
2. Blend until smooth and creamy.
3. Pour into glasses and garnish with mint leaves if desired.
4. Serve immediately.

Nutrition: Calories: 190; Fat: 2g; Carbs: 37g; Protein: 8g; Sugar: 20g; Fiber: 5g;

Equipment: Blender; Measuring cups; Measuring spoons.

Golden Turmeric and Pineapple Smoothie

Prep time: 7 min
Cook time: 0 min
Total time: 7 min
Servings: 2

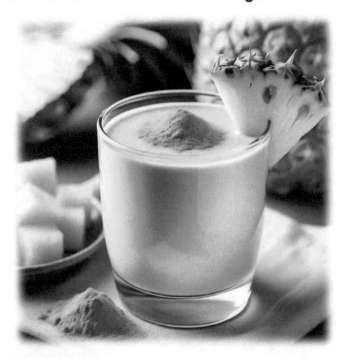

Ingredients:

- ✓ Fresh pineapple chunks, 1 cup
- ✓ Greek yogurt, 1 cup
- ✓ Turmeric powder, 1 tsp
- ✓ Honey, 2 tbsp
- ✓ Water, 1/2 cup
- ✓ Black pepper, a pinch
- ✓ Ice cubes, 1/2 cup (optional)

Directions:

1. In a blender, combine fresh pineapple chunks, Greek yogurt, turmeric powder, honey, black pepper, and water.
2. Add ice cubes if a colder smoothie is desired.
3. Blend until smooth and creamy.
4. Pour into glasses and serve immediately.

Nutrition: Calories: 210; Fat: 3g; Carbs: 43g; Protein: 7g; Sugar: 32g; Fiber: 2g;

Equipment: Blender; Measuring cups; Measuring spoons.

Creamy Papaya and Spinach Smoothie

Prep time: 7 min
Cook time: 0 min
Total time: 7 min
Servings: 2

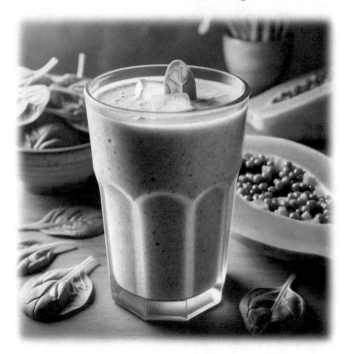

Ingredients:

- ✓ Papaya, peeled and deseeded, 1 cup
- ✓ Fresh spinach, 2 cups
- ✓ Greek yogurt, 1 cup
- ✓ Honey, 2 tbsp
- ✓ Water, 1/2 cup
- ✓ Ice cubes, 1/2 cup (optional)

Directions:

1. In a blender, combine the papaya, fresh spinach, Greek yogurt, honey, and water.
2. Add ice cubes if a colder smoothie is desired.
3. Blend until smooth and creamy.
4. Pour into glasses and serve immediately.

Nutrition: Calories: 190; Fat: 3g; Carbs: 38g; Protein: 6g; Sugar: 30g; Fiber: 4g;

Equipment: Blender; Measuring cups; Measuring spoons.

SALAD RECIPES

Crisp Cucumber Salad with Dill Vinaigrette

Prep time: 10 min   **Total time:** 10 min
Cook time: 0 min   **Servings:** 4

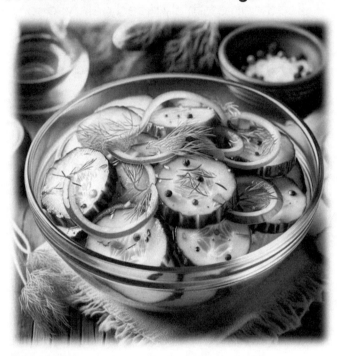

Ingredients:

✓ Cucumbers, thinly sliced, 2 cups
✓ Red onion, thinly sliced, 1/4 cup
✓ Fresh dill, chopped, 2 tbsp
✓ Olive oil, 3 tbsp
✓ White wine vinegar, 1 tbsp
✓ Salt, 1 pinch
✓ Black pepper, 1 pinch

Directions:

1. In a large salad bowl, combine the thinly sliced cucumbers and red onion.
2. In a small bowl, whisk together the olive oil, white wine vinegar, chopped dill, salt, and black pepper to create the vinaigrette.
3. Drizzle the vinaigrette over the cucumber and red onion mixture.

4. Toss gently until all ingredients are well combined.
5. Refrigerate for about 30 minutes before serving for flavors to meld.

Nutrition: Calories: 110; Fat: 10g; Carbs: 4g; Protein: 1g; Sugar: 2g; Fiber: 1g;

Equipment: Large salad bowl; Small mixing bowl; Whisk; Knife; Measuring cups; Measuring spoons.

Tomato and Red Onion Salad with Cilantro

Prep time: 10 min   **Total time:** 10 min
Cook time: 0 min   **Servings:** 4

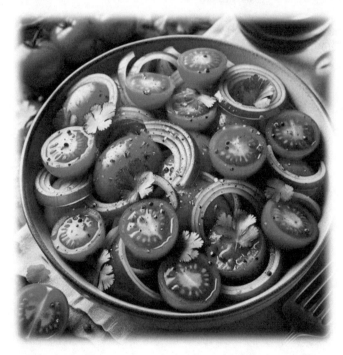

Ingredients:

✓ Cherry tomatoes, halved, 2 cups
✓ Red onion, thinly sliced, 1/2 cup
✓ Fresh cilantro, chopped, 3 tbsp
✓ Olive oil, 2 tbsp
✓ White wine vinegar, 1 tbsp
✓ Salt, 1 pinch
✓ Black pepper, 1 pinch

Directions:

1. In a large salad bowl, combine the halved cherry tomatoes and thinly sliced red onion.
2. Sprinkle the fresh cilantro over the tomato and onion mixture.
3. In a small bowl, whisk together the olive oil, white wine vinegar, salt, and black pepper to create a dressing.
4. Drizzle the dressing over the tomato, onion, and cilantro mixture.
5. Toss gently until all ingredients are well combined.
6. Serve immediately or refrigerate for later use.

Nutrition: Calories: 90; Fat: 7g; Carbs: 6g; Protein: 1g; Sugar: 4g; Fiber: 1g;

Equipment: Large salad bowl; Small mixing bowl; Whisk; Knife; Measuring cups; Measuring spoons.

Apple and Celery Salad with Walnuts

Prep time: 15 min   **Total time:** 15 min
Cook time: 0 min   **Servings:** 4

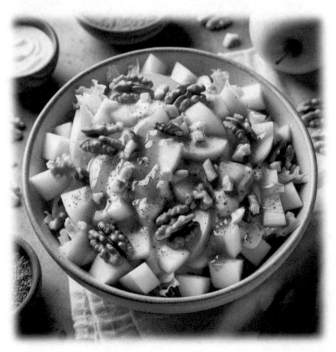

Ingredients:

✓ Fresh apples, diced, 2 pcs
✓ Celery, thinly sliced, 1 cup
✓ Toasted walnuts, 1 cup
✓ Greek yogurt, 1/2 cup
✓ Honey, 1 tbsp
✓ Salt, 1 pinch
✓ Black pepper, 1 pinch

Directions:

1. In a large salad bowl, combine the diced apples, thinly sliced celery, and toasted walnuts.
2. In a separate small bowl, whisk together the Greek yogurt, honey, salt, and black pepper to make the dressing.
3. Pour the dressing over the apple mixture and toss gently to coat all the ingredients.
4. Serve immediately or refrigerate for later use.

Nutrition: Calories: 220; Fat: 15g; Carbs: 20g; Protein: 4g; Sugar: 12g; Fiber: 3g;

Equipment: Large salad bowl; Small mixing bowl; Whisk; Knife; Measuring cups; Measuring spoons.

Mixed Bean Salad with Parsley and Feta

Prep time: 15 min   **Total time:** 15 min
Cook time: 0 min   **Servings:** 4

Ingredients:

✓ Canned baked beans, drained and rinsed, 2 cups
✓ Cherry tomatoes, halved, 1 cup
✓ Chopped fresh parsley, 2 tbsp
✓ Red onion, thinly sliced, 1/2 cup
✓ Feta cheese, crumbled, 1 cup
✓ Olive oil, 2 tbsp
✓ White wine vinegar, 1 tbsp
✓ Salt, 1 pinch
✓ Black pepper, 1 pinch

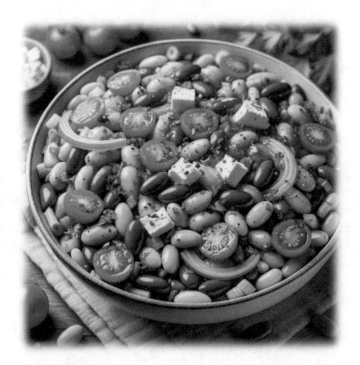

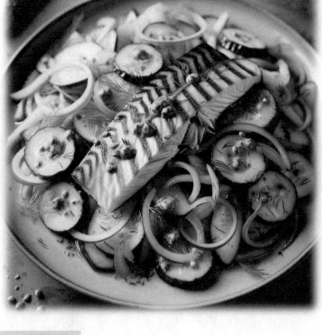

Directions:

1. In a large salad bowl, combine the drained and rinsed beans, halved cherry tomatoes, chopped parsley, and thinly sliced red onion.
2. In a separate small bowl, whisk together the olive oil, white wine vinegar, salt, and black pepper to create the dressing.
3. Pour the dressing over the bean mixture and toss gently to coat all ingredients evenly.
4. Top with crumbled feta cheese.
5. Serve immediately or refrigerate for later use.

Nutrition: Calories: 230; Fat: 10g; Carbs: 25g; Protein: 8g; Sugar: 3g; Fiber: 7g;

Equipment: Large salad bowl; Small mixing bowl; Whisk; Knife; Measuring cups; Measuring spoons.

Mackerel and Cucumber Slaw with Dijon Dressing

Prep time: 20 min   **Total time:** 20 min
Cook time: 0 min   **Servings:** 4

Ingredients:

- ✓ Fresh mackerel fillets, grilled and flaked, 4 pcs
- ✓ Cucumbers, thinly sliced, 2 cups
- ✓ Red onion, thinly sliced, 1/2 cup
- ✓ Olive oil, 2 tbsp
- ✓ White wine vinegar, 1 tbsp
- ✓ Dijon mustard, 2 tsp
- ✓ Honey, 1 tbsp
- ✓ Salt, 1 pinch
- ✓ Black pepper, 1 pinch
- ✓ Fresh dill, chopped, 1 tbsp

Directions:

1. In a large mixing bowl, combine the thinly sliced cucumbers and red onion.
2. In a separate smaller bowl, whisk together olive oil, white wine vinegar, Dijon mustard, honey, salt, and black pepper to create the Dijon dressing.
3. Pour the dressing over the cucumber and onion mix and toss gently to coat.
4. Gently fold in the grilled and flaked mackerel pieces.
5. Garnish with chopped fresh dill.
6. Serve immediately or refrigerate for later use.

Nutrition: Calories: 260; Fat: 14g; Carbs: 10g; Protein: 24g; Sugar: 4g; Fiber: 1g;

Equipment: Large mixing bowl; Small mixing bowl; Whisk; Knife; Measuring cups; Measuring spoons.

Herring and Beetroot Salad with Fresh Dill

Prep time: 20 min
Cook time: 0 min

Total time: 20 min
Servings: 4

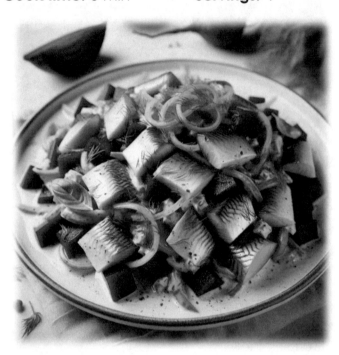

Ingredients:

- ✓ Fresh herring fillets, marinated and chopped, 4 pcs
- ✓ Beetroots, cooked and diced, 2 cups
- ✓ Red onion, thinly sliced, 1/2 cup
- ✓ Fresh dill, chopped, 2 tbsp
- ✓ Greek yogurt, 1 cup
- ✓ Olive oil, 1 tbsp
- ✓ White wine vinegar, 1 tbsp
- ✓ Salt, 1 pinch
- ✓ Black pepper, 1 pinch

Directions:

1. In a large mixing bowl, combine diced beetroots, chopped herring fillets, and thinly sliced red onion.
2. In a separate smaller bowl, whisk together Greek yogurt, olive oil, white wine vinegar, salt, and black pepper to create the dressing.
3. Pour the dressing over the beetroot and herring mix and toss gently to coat.
4. Garnish with chopped fresh dill.
5. Serve immediately or refrigerate for later use.

Nutrition: Calories: 220; Fat: 9g; Carbs: 16g; Protein: 19g; Sugar: 12g; Fiber: 4g;

Equipment: Large mixing bowl; Small mixing bowl; Whisk; Knife; Measuring cups; Measuring spoons.

Grilled Chicken and Peach Salad with Honey Vinaigrette

Prep time: 20 min
Cook time: 15 min

Total time: 35 min
Servings: 4

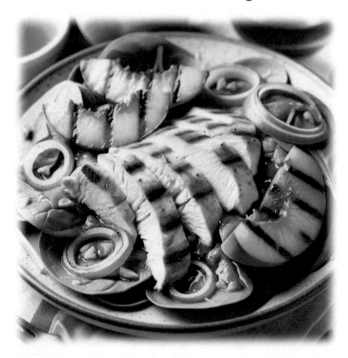

Ingredients:

- ✓ Grilled chicken breasts, sliced, 4 pcs
- ✓ Fresh peaches, halved and pitted, 4 pcs
- ✓ Fresh spinach, 4 cups
- ✓ Red onion, thinly sliced, 1/2 cup
- ✓ Olive oil, 3 tbsp
- ✓ White wine vinegar, 1 tbsp
- ✓ Honey, 2 tbsp
- ✓ Salt, 1 pinch

✓ Black pepper, 1 pinch

Directions:

1. Preheat the grill to medium heat.
2. Grill the chicken breasts until fully cooked, approximately 7 minutes per side. Once cooked, let them rest for a few minutes before slicing.
3. Place peaches, cut-side down, on the grill. Grill for about 3-4 minutes until they have grill marks and are slightly softened.
4. In a small bowl, whisk together olive oil, white wine vinegar, honey, salt, and black pepper to make the vinaigrette.
5. In a large salad bowl, combine fresh spinach, sliced grilled chicken, grilled peaches, and thinly sliced red onion.
6. Drizzle the honey vinaigrette over the salad and toss to combine.
7. Serve immediately.

Nutrition: Calories: 320; Fat: 12g; Carbs: 20g; Protein: 32g; Sugar: 15g; Fiber: 3g;

Equipment: Grill; Small bowl; Whisk; Knife; Large salad bowl; Measuring cups; Measuring spoons.

Spiced Turkey and Grape Salad with Feta Crumbles

Prep time: 15 min
Cook time: 15 min
Total time: 30 min
Servings: 4

Ingredients:

✓ Ground turkey, 1 lb
✓ Red grapes, 2 cups
✓ Fresh spinach, 4 cups
✓ Feta cheese, crumbled, 1 cup
✓ Olive oil, 2 tbsp
✓ Dijon mustard, 1 tsp
✓ Honey, 1 tbsp
✓ White wine vinegar, 2 tbsp
✓ Salt, 1 pinch
✓ Black pepper, 1 pinch
✓ Cinnamon, 1/2 tsp
✓ Turmeric powder, 1/2 tsp

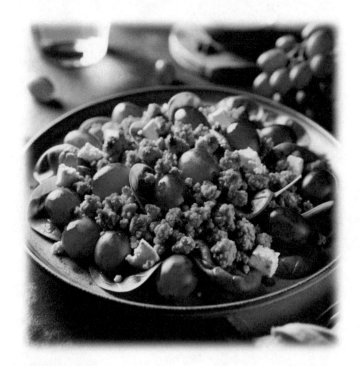

Directions:

1. In a large skillet, heat 1 tbsp olive oil over medium heat. Add ground turkey, salt, black pepper, cinnamon, and turmeric. Cook until the turkey is browned and fully cooked through.
2. In a small bowl, whisk together the remaining olive oil, Dijon mustard, honey, and white wine vinegar to make the dressing.
3. In a large salad bowl, combine fresh spinach, cooked spiced turkey, grapes, and crumbled feta cheese.
4. Drizzle the dressing over the salad and toss gently to combine.
5. Serve immediately.

Nutrition: Calories: 340; Fat: 17g; Carbs: 20g; Protein: 28g; Sugar: 12g; Fiber: 2g;

Equipment: Large skillet; Small bowl; Whisk; Large salad bowl; Measuring cups; Measuring spoons.

Broccoli and Cauliflower Salad with Lemon Zest

Prep time: 15 min
Cook time: 0 min
Total time: 15 min
Servings: 4

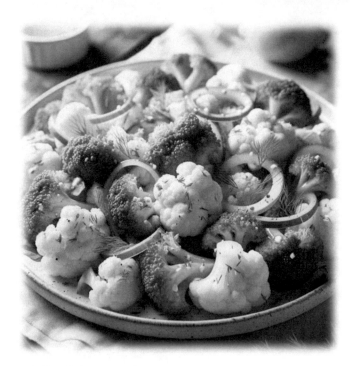

Ingredients:

- ✓ Broccoli, 4 cups
- ✓ Cauliflower, 4 cups
- ✓ Olive oil, 2 tbsp
- ✓ Lemon zest, from 1 lemon
- ✓ Salt, 1 pinch
- ✓ Black pepper, 1 pinch
- ✓ Fresh dill, chopped, 2 tbsp
- ✓ Greek yogurt, 1/2 cup
- ✓ Honey, 1 tbsp
- ✓ Red onion, thinly sliced, 1/2 cup

Directions:

1. In a large bowl, combine broccoli and cauliflower.
2. In a separate small bowl, whisk together olive oil, lemon zest, salt, black pepper, Greek yogurt, and honey until well combined.
3. Pour the dressing over the broccoli and cauliflower and toss to coat.
4. Add in the red onion and fresh dill, and toss again.
5. Serve chilled.

Nutrition: Calories: 140; Fat: 7g; Carbs: 15g; Protein: 6g; Sugar: 6g; Fiber: 4g;

Equipment: Large bowl; Small bowl; Whisk; Measuring cups; Measuring spoons; Zester.

Charred Green Bean Salad with Garlic Aioli

Prep time: 10 min   **Total time:** 20 min
Cook time: 10 min   **Servings:** 4

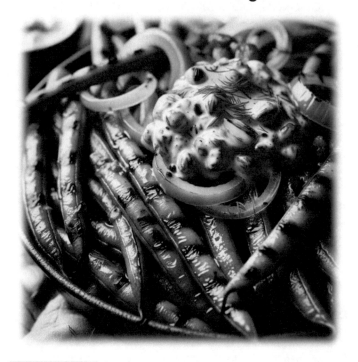

Ingredients:

- ✓ Green beans, 4 cups
- ✓ Olive oil, 2 tbsp
- ✓ Salt, 1 pinch
- ✓ Black pepper, 1 pinch
- ✓ Garlic cloves, 2, minced
- ✓ Greek yogurt, 1/2 cup
- ✓ Lemon zest, from 1 lemon
- ✓ Dijon mustard, 1 tsp
- ✓ Fresh dill, chopped, 2 tbsp
- ✓ Red onion, thinly sliced, 1/2 cup

Directions:

1. Preheat the grill or a grill pan over medium-high heat.
2. Toss the green beans with olive oil, salt, and black pepper.
3. Place the green beans on the grill and cook, turning occasionally, until charred and tender, about 8-10 minutes.
4. For the aioli, in a small bowl, mix together the minced garlic, Greek yogurt, lemon zest, and Dijon mustard until smooth.

5. Once the green beans are done, transfer them to a serving plate.
6. Drizzle with the garlic aioli, then sprinkle with fresh dill and red onion.
7. Serve immediately.

Nutrition: Calories: 120; Fat: 6g; Carbs: 12g; Protein: 5g; Sugar: 4g; Fiber: 3g;

Equipment: Grill or grill pan; Mixing bowl; Tongs; Measuring cups; Measuring spoons.

Smoked Salmon and Fennel Salad with Citrus Vinaigrette

Prep time: 15 min   **Total time:** 15 min
Cook time: 0 min   **Servings:** 4

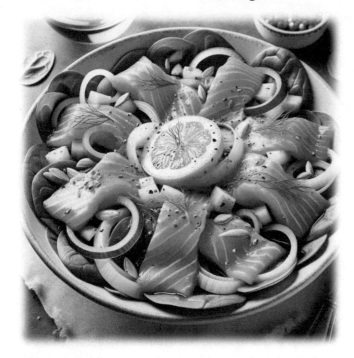

Ingredients:

✓ Smoked salmon, 8 oz, thinly sliced
✓ Fennel bulb, 1, thinly sliced
✓ Fresh spinach, 4 cups
✓ Red onion, thinly sliced, 1/2 cup
✓ Olive oil, 3 tbsp
✓ White wine vinegar, 2 tbsp
✓ Honey, 1 tbsp
✓ Lemon zest, from 1 lemon
✓ Salt, 1 pinch
✓ Black pepper, 1 pinch
✓ Garlic cloves, 1, minced

Directions:

1. In a large salad bowl, combine smoked salmon, thinly sliced fennel bulb, fresh spinach, and red onion.
2. In a small mixing bowl, whisk together olive oil, white wine vinegar, honey, minced garlic, and lemon zest until well combined.
3. Season the vinaigrette with salt and black pepper.
4. Drizzle the vinaigrette over the salad and gently toss to combine.
5. Serve immediately.

Nutrition: Calories: 210; Fat: 13g; Carbs: 10g; Protein: 12g; Sugar: 4g; Fiber: 3g;

Equipment: Large salad bowl; Small mixing bowl; Whisk; Measuring cups; Measuring spoons.

Beef Strip and Roasted Brussels Sprouts Salad

Prep time: 10 min   **Total time:** 25 min
Cook time: 15 min   **Servings:** 4

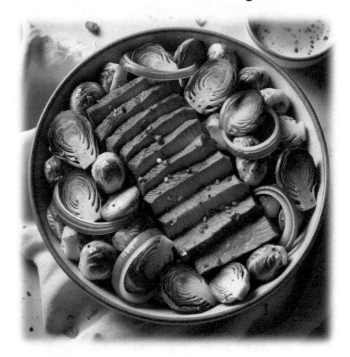

Ingredients:

✓ Beef strip steak, 16 oz

- ✓ Brussels sprouts, 2 cups, halved
- ✓ Olive oil, 2 tbsp
- ✓ Red onion, thinly sliced, 1/2 cup
- ✓ Salt, 1 pinch
- ✓ Black pepper, 1 pinch
- ✓ Garlic cloves, 2, minced
- ✓ Lemon zest, from 1 lemon
- ✓ White wine vinegar, 1 tbsp
- ✓ Chopped fresh parsley, 2 tbsp

Directions:

1. Preheat oven to 425°F (220°C).
2. In a large mixing bowl, toss Brussels sprouts with 1 tbsp olive oil, salt, and black pepper. Place on a baking sheet and roast in the oven for 12-15 minutes or until tender and lightly browned.
3. While the Brussels sprouts are roasting, heat 1 tbsp olive oil in a skillet over medium-high heat. Season the beef strip steak with salt and black pepper. Once the skillet is hot, add the beef strip steak and cook for 3-4 minutes on each side or until desired doneness. Remove from the skillet and let rest for a few minutes before slicing thinly.
4. In a small mixing bowl, whisk together minced garlic, lemon zest, white wine vinegar, and chopped parsley to create the dressing.
5. In a large salad bowl, combine roasted Brussels sprouts, thinly sliced beef, and red onion. Drizzle with the dressing and gently toss to combine.
6. Serve immediately.

Nutrition: Calories: 330; Fat: 20g; Carbs: 10g; Protein: 28g; Sugar: 3g; Fiber: 4g;

Equipment: Oven; Large mixing bowl; Baking sheet; Skillet; Small mixing bowl; Salad bowl.

Warm Lentil and Spinach Salad with Poached Eggs

Prep time: 10 min
Cook time: 20 min
Total time: 30 min
Servings: 4

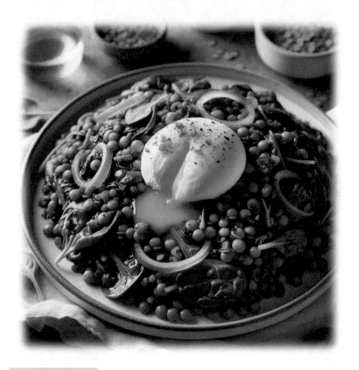

Ingredients:

- ✓ Dried green lentils, 1 cup
- ✓ Fresh spinach, 4 cups
- ✓ Eggs, 4 pcs
- ✓ Olive oil, 2 tbsp
- ✓ Garlic cloves, 2, minced
- ✓ Red onion, thinly sliced, 1/2 cup
- ✓ Dijon mustard, 1 tsp
- ✓ White wine vinegar, 2 tbsp
- ✓ Salt, 1 pinch
- ✓ Black pepper, 1 pinch
- ✓ Water, 4 cups (for poaching eggs)

Directions:

1. Rinse lentils under cold water. In a medium pot, bring 3 cups of water to a boil, add lentils, reduce the heat, and simmer for 15-20 minutes or until tender. Drain.
2. While lentils are cooking, heat 1 tbsp olive oil in a skillet over medium heat. Add the minced garlic and thinly sliced red onion. Sauté for 2-3 minutes or until onion is translucent.
3. Add fresh spinach to the skillet and cook just until wilted. Transfer spinach mixture to a large mixing bowl.
4. In a separate small bowl, whisk together 1 tbsp olive oil, Dijon mustard, white wine

vinegar, salt, and black pepper to create the dressing.

5. Add cooked lentils to the spinach mixture. Drizzle with the dressing and toss to combine.

6. Bring 4 cups of water to a light simmer in a deep skillet. Crack one egg into a small bowl and gently slide it into the simmering water. Repeat with the remaining eggs. Poach for 3-4 minutes or until whites are set but yolks remain runny. Use a slotted spoon to transfer eggs to a paper towel to drain.

7. Divide the lentil and spinach salad among plates and top with a poached egg.

Nutrition: Calories: 250; Fat: 10g; Carbs: 28g; Protein: 12g; Sugar: 3g; Fiber: 6g;

Equipment: Medium pot; Skillet; Large mixing bowl; Small mixing bowl; Slotted spoon.

Roasted Butternut Squash and Quinoa Salad with Cranberries

Prep time: 15 min
Cook time: 30 min

Total time: 45 min
Servings: 4

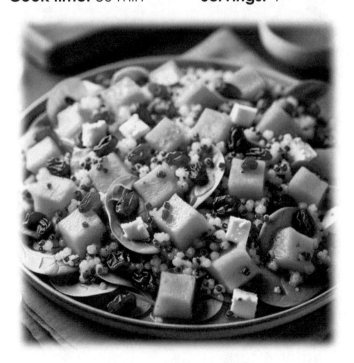

Ingredients:

- ✓ Butternut squash, peeled, seeded and diced, 2 cups
- ✓ Quinoa, rinsed and drained, 1 cup
- ✓ Dried cranberries, 1/2 cup
- ✓ Olive oil, 2 tbsp
- ✓ Fresh spinach, 2 cups
- ✓ Feta cheese, crumbled, 1/2 cup
- ✓ Honey, 1 tbsp
- ✓ White wine vinegar, 1 tbsp
- ✓ Dijon mustard, 1 tsp
- ✓ Salt, 1 pinch
- ✓ Black pepper, 1 pinch
- ✓ Chopped fresh parsley, 1 tbsp
- ✓ Water, 2 cups

Directions:

1. Preheat oven to 400°F (205°C). Spread diced butternut squash on a baking sheet, drizzle with 1 tbsp olive oil, and season with salt and pepper. Roast for 20-25 minutes or until tender and slightly caramelized.

2. In a medium pot, bring 2 cups of water to a boil. Add quinoa and a pinch of salt, reduce heat, cover, and simmer for 15 minutes or until quinoa is cooked and water is absorbed. Fluff with a fork and set aside.

3. In a large mixing bowl, combine roasted butternut squash, cooked quinoa, dried cranberries, fresh spinach, and feta cheese.

4. In a small bowl, whisk together 1 tbsp olive oil, honey, white wine vinegar, Dijon mustard, salt, and black pepper to create the dressing.

5. Pour the dressing over the salad and toss gently to combine. Garnish with chopped fresh parsley.

Nutrition: Calories: 340; Fat: 12g; Carbs: 52g; Protein: 9g; Sugar: 14g; Fiber: 7g;

Equipment: Baking sheet; Medium pot; Large mixing bowl; Small mixing bowl.

SOUP RECIPES

Fresh Herb and Cabbage Broth

Prep time: 10 min **Total time:** 35 min
Cook time: 25 min **Servings:** 4

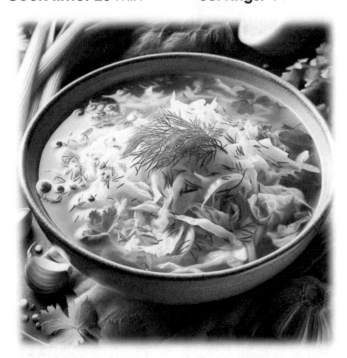

Ingredients:

✓ Green cabbage, shredded, 2 cups
✓ Fresh dill, chopped, 2 tbsp
✓ Fresh cilantro, chopped, 2 tbsp
✓ Garlic cloves, minced, 2 pcs
✓ Celery, thinly sliced, 1 cup
✓ Olive oil, 1 tbsp
✓ Water, 6 cups
✓ Salt, 1 pinch
✓ Black pepper, 1 pinch
✓ Lemon zest, 1 lemon

Directions:

1. In a large pot, heat olive oil over medium heat. Add the minced garlic and thinly sliced celery. Sauté for 2-3 minutes until they start to soften.
2. Add the shredded green cabbage to the pot and continue to sauté for

another 5 minutes until the cabbage starts to wilt.
3. Pour in the water and bring the mixture to a boil. Once boiling, reduce the heat and let it simmer for 15 minutes.
4. Add the fresh dill, fresh cilantro, salt, and black pepper. Let it simmer for another 5 minutes.
5. Turn off the heat and add the lemon zest. Stir well.
6. Serve the broth warm, garnished with additional fresh herbs if desired.

Nutrition: Calories: 50; Fat: 3g; Carbs: 7g; Protein: 1g; Sugar: 2g; Fiber: 3g;

Equipment: Large pot.

Tilapia Soup with Green Peas

Prep time: 15 min **Total time:** 35 min
Cook time: 20 min **Servings:** 4

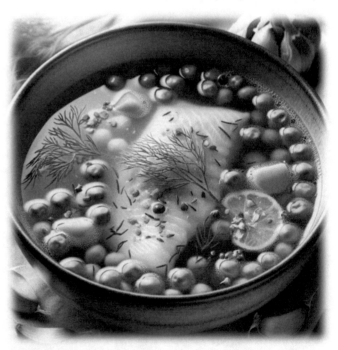

Ingredients:

✓ Tilapia fillets, 4 pcs (6 oz each)
✓ Green peas, frozen or fresh, 2 cups
✓ Garlic cloves, minced, 3 pcs
✓ Olive oil, 2 tbsp
✓ Water, 6 cups
✓ Salt, 1 pinch

- ✓ Black pepper, 1 pinch
- ✓ Fresh dill, chopped, 1 tbsp
- ✓ Lemon zest, from 1 lemon

Directions:

1. In a large pot, heat olive oil over medium heat. Add the minced garlic and sauté until fragrant.
2. Add the tilapia fillets to the pot and cook each side for about 3-4 minutes until they turn opaque.
3. Pour in the water and bring the mixture to a gentle boil. Once boiling, reduce the heat to low.
4. Add the green peas to the pot and let it simmer for 10 minutes.
5. Season the soup with salt, black pepper, and fresh dill.
6. Turn off the heat and add the lemon zest. Stir well.
7. Serve the soup hot, garnished with additional fresh dill if desired.

Nutrition: Calories: 210; Fat: 7g; Carbs: 12g; Protein: 28g; Sugar: 4g; Fiber: 4g;

Equipment: Large pot.

Chicken and Barley Herb Soup

Prep time: 20 min   **Total time:** 60 min
Cook time: 40 min   **Servings:** 4

Ingredients:

- ✓ Grilled chicken breasts, sliced, 4 pcs
- ✓ Barley, 1 cup
- ✓ Celery, thinly sliced, 1 cup
- ✓ Garlic cloves, minced, 2 pcs
- ✓ Olive oil, 2 tbsp
- ✓ Water, 8 cups
- ✓ Salt, 1 pinch
- ✓ Black pepper, 1 pinch
- ✓ Chopped fresh parsley, 2 tbsp
- ✓ Fresh dill, chopped, 1 tbsp

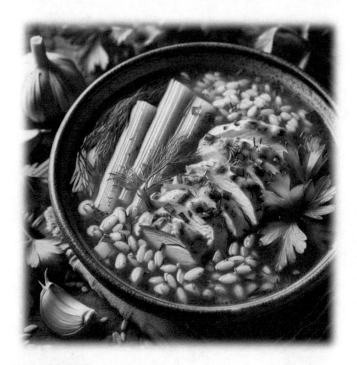

Directions:

1. In a large pot, heat the olive oil over medium heat. Add the minced garlic and sauté until fragrant.
2. Add the thinly sliced celery to the pot and cook for about 3 minutes until slightly softened.
3. Pour in the water and bring the mixture to a boil.
4. Once boiling, add the barley and reduce the heat to low. Let it simmer for 20 minutes.
5. Add the sliced grilled chicken breasts to the pot and continue to simmer for another 10 minutes or until the barley is tender.
6. Season the soup with salt, black pepper, chopped fresh parsley, and fresh dill.
7. Serve the soup hot, garnished with additional fresh herbs if desired.

Nutrition: Calories: 260; Fat: 8g; Carbs: 25g; Protein: 20g; Sugar: 2g; Fiber: 4g;

Equipment: Large pot.

Moroccan Spiced Lentil and Vegetable Soup

Prep time: 15 min   **Total time:** 60 min
Cook time: 45 min   **Servings:** 6

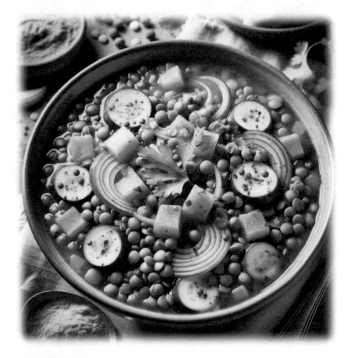

Ingredients:

- ✓ Dried green lentils, 1 cup
- ✓ Olive oil, 2 tbsp
- ✓ Garlic cloves, minced, 3 pcs
- ✓ Red onion, thinly sliced, 1 cup
- ✓ Celery, thinly sliced, 1 cup
- ✓ Zucchini, thinly sliced, 2 cups
- ✓ Carrot, grated, 2 cups (not in main table, added for flavor)
- ✓ Butternut squash, peeled, seeded and diced, 2 cups
- ✓ Turmeric powder, 1 tsp
- ✓ Cinnamon, 0.5 tsp
- ✓ Salt, 1 pinch
- ✓ Black pepper, 1 pinch
- ✓ Water, 8 cups
- ✓ Chopped fresh parsley, for garnish, 2 tbsp
- ✓ Fresh cilantro, chopped, for garnish, 2 tbsp

Directions:

1. In a large pot, heat olive oil over medium heat. Add the minced garlic and thinly sliced red onion. Sauté until the onion becomes translucent.
2. Stir in the celery and zucchini. Cook for another 3-4 minutes until softened.
3. Add the grated carrot and diced butternut squash to the pot. Sprinkle in the turmeric, cinnamon, salt, and black pepper. Stir well to combine.
4. Pour in the dried green lentils followed by water. Bring the mixture to a boil.
5. Reduce the heat and let the soup simmer for about 35-40 minutes, or until the lentils are tender.
6. Taste and adjust seasonings as needed.
7. Serve hot, garnished with chopped fresh parsley and fresh cilantro.

Nutrition: Calories: 210; Fat: 5g; Carbs: 35g; Protein: 10g; Sugar: 4g; Fiber: 9g;

Equipment: Large pot.

Turkey Meatball and Spinach Soup

Prep time: 20 min   **Total time:** 50 min
Cook time: 30 min   **Servings:** 6

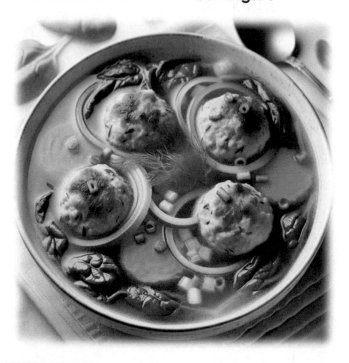

Ingredients:

- ✓ Ground turkey, 1 lb
- ✓ Fresh spinach, 3 cups
- ✓ Garlic cloves, minced, 3 pcs

- ✓ Eggs, 1 pc
- ✓ Salt, 1 pinch
- ✓ Black pepper, 1 pinch
- ✓ Olive oil, 2 tbsp
- ✓ Red onion, thinly sliced, 1 cup
- ✓ Celery, thinly sliced, 1 cup
- ✓ Carrot, thinly sliced, 1 cup
- ✓ Water, 6 cups
- ✓ Fresh dill, chopped, 2 tbsp for garnish

Directions:

1. In a mixing bowl, combine ground turkey, minced garlic, egg, salt, and black pepper. Mix until well combined.
2. Shape the mixture into small meatballs, around 1 inch in diameter.
3. In a large pot, heat olive oil over medium heat. Add the thinly sliced red onion and sauté until translucent.
4. Add the celery and carrot to the pot, and cook for another 5 minutes.
5. Gently place the turkey meatballs into the pot. Pour in water and bring to a boil.
6. Reduce heat and let it simmer for 20 minutes.
7. Stir in the fresh spinach and cook for an additional 3-4 minutes until wilted.
8. Taste and adjust seasonings as needed.
9. Serve hot, garnished with fresh dill.

Nutrition: Calories: 220; Fat: 8g; Carbs: 10g; Protein: 28g; Sugar: 3g; Fiber: 2g;

Equipment: Large pot; Mixing bowl.

Rustic Mushroom and Thyme Soup

Prep time: 15 min
Cook time: 35 min

Total time: 50 min
Servings: 4

Ingredients:

- ✓ Portobello mushrooms, 4 large caps
- ✓ Garlic cloves, minced, 4 pcs
- ✓ Olive oil, 3 tbsp
- ✓ Red onion, thinly sliced, 1 cup
- ✓ Celery, thinly sliced, 1 cup
- ✓ Carrot, thinly sliced, 1 cup
- ✓ Water, 4 cups
- ✓ Fresh thyme, 1 tbsp (chopped, plus extra for garnish)
- ✓ Salt, 1 pinch
- ✓ Black pepper, 1 pinch

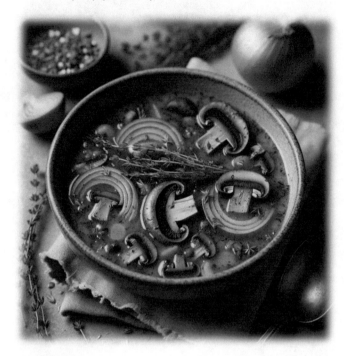

Directions:

1. Clean the Portobello mushrooms with a damp cloth and chop them into bite-sized pieces.
2. In a large pot, heat olive oil over medium heat. Add the minced garlic and thinly sliced red onion. Sauté until the onion is translucent.
3. Add the celery and grated carrot, and cook for another 5 minutes.
4. Stir in the chopped mushrooms and sauté until they release their juices and become tender.
5. Pour in the water and bring to a boil.
6. Reduce heat, add fresh thyme, salt, and black pepper. Let it simmer for 25 minutes.
7. Taste and adjust the seasoning if necessary.
8. Serve hot, garnished with extra thyme.

Nutrition: Calories: 140; Fat: 7g; Carbs: 15g; Protein: 5g; Sugar: 3g; Fiber: 3g;

Equipment: Large pot; Knife; Chopping board.

Mediterranean Sea Bass Soup

Prep time: 20 min   **Total time:** 60 min
Cook time: 40 min   **Servings:** 4

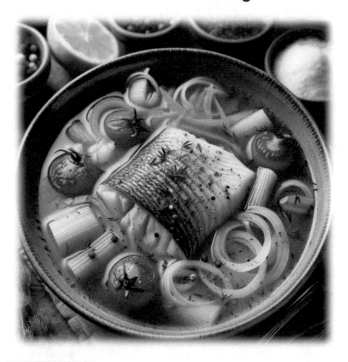

4. Add the cherry tomatoes and let them soften for about 5 minutes.
5. Pour in the water, followed by the fresh thyme and dill.
6. Carefully place the sea bass fillets in the soup. Let it simmer gently until the fish is cooked through, about 15 minutes.
7. Adjust the seasoning if needed and add lemon zest.
8. Serve hot, garnished with additional dill if desired.

Nutrition: Calories: 220; Fat: 9g; Carbs: 10g; Protein: 25g; Sugar: 4g; Fiber: 3g;

Equipment: Large pot; Knife; Chopping board; Zester.

Ingredients:

- ✓ Sea bass fillets, 4 oz each
- ✓ Olive oil, 3 tbsp
- ✓ Garlic cloves, minced, 3 pcs
- ✓ Red onion, thinly sliced, 1 cup
- ✓ Celery, thinly sliced, 1 cup
- ✓ Carrot, grated, 1 cup
- ✓ Cherry tomatoes, 2 cups
- ✓ Fresh thyme (chopped), 1 tbsp
- ✓ Fresh dill, chopped, 2 tbsp
- ✓ Black pepper, 1 pinch
- ✓ Salt, 1 pinch
- ✓ Water, 5 cups
- ✓ Lemon zest, 1 lemon

Directions:

1. Season the sea bass fillets with salt and black pepper.
2. In a large pot, heat olive oil over medium heat. Add minced garlic and thinly sliced red onion. Sauté until the onion is translucent.
3. Add the thinly sliced celery and grated carrot to the pot and cook for another 5 minutes.

GOULASH RECIPES

Tofu and Mushroom Goulash in Tomato Sauce

Prep time: 15 min
Cook time: 30 min
Total time: 45 min
Servings: 4

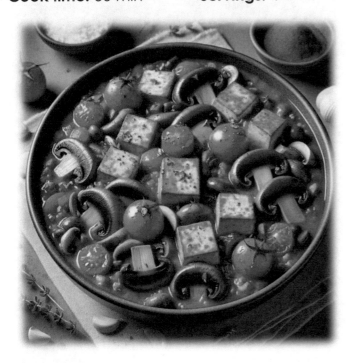

Ingredients:

✓ Firm tofu, cubed, 14 oz
✓ Portobello mushrooms, 4 large caps, sliced
✓ Olive oil, 2 tbsp
✓ Garlic cloves, minced, 3 pcs
✓ Red onion, thinly sliced, 1 cup
✓ Cherry tomatoes, 2 cups
✓ Fresh thyme (chopped), 1 tbsp
✓ Fresh dill, chopped, 1 tbsp
✓ Black pepper, 1 pinch
✓ Salt, 1 pinch
✓ Water, 2 cups
✓ Paprika, 1 tsp

Directions:

1. Press the tofu cubes to remove excess moisture.
2. In a large pan, heat olive oil over medium heat. Add minced garlic and thinly sliced red onion. Sauté until the onion is translucent.
3. Add the sliced Portobello mushrooms and sauté for another 5-7 minutes, until they release their juices.
4. Add the cherry tomatoes, cubed tofu, and spices (paprika, salt, and black pepper). Stir well.
5. Add water, then bring the mixture to a boil. Reduce heat to a simmer.
6. Cover and let simmer for 20 minutes, stirring occasionally.
7. Adjust seasoning if needed, and stir in fresh thyme and dill.
8. Serve hot, garnished with more dill if desired.

Nutrition: Calories: 210; Fat: 9g; Carbs: 14g; Protein: 18g; Sugar: 5g; Fiber: 4g;

Equipment: Large pan; Knife; Chopping board.

Chickpea and Vegetable Goulash

Prep time: 20 min
Cook time: 40 min
Total time: 60 min
Servings: 4

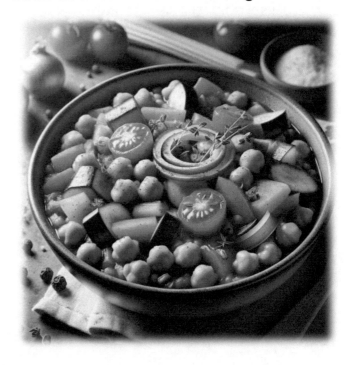

Ingredients:

- ✓ Chickpeas, cooked, 2 cups
- ✓ Olive oil, 2 tbsp
- ✓ Garlic cloves, minced, 3 pcs
- ✓ Red onion, thinly sliced, 1 cup
- ✓ Celery, thinly sliced, 1 cup
- ✓ Carrot, diced, 1 cup
- ✓ Zucchini, diced, 1 cup
- ✓ Cherry tomatoes, 1.5 cups
- ✓ Paprika, 1 tsp
- ✓ Black pepper, 1 pinch
- ✓ Salt, 1 pinch
- ✓ Water, 2.5 cups
- ✓ Fresh thyme (chopped), 1 tbsp
- ✓ Fresh cilantro, chopped, 1 tbsp

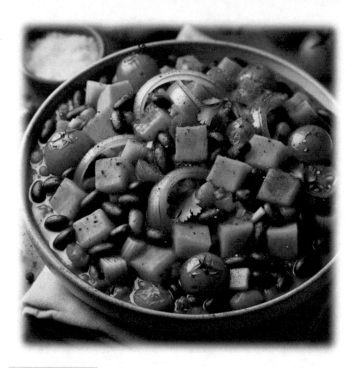

Directions:

1. In a large pot, heat olive oil over medium heat. Add minced garlic and thinly sliced red onion, sauté until translucent.
2. Add thinly sliced celery, diced carrot, and diced zucchini. Continue sautéing for another 5-7 minutes.
3. Stir in the chickpeas, cherry tomatoes, paprika, salt, and black pepper. Mix well.
4. Pour in the water and bring to a boil. Once boiling, reduce the heat to low and let it simmer for about 30 minutes.
5. Near the end of cooking, stir in the fresh thyme and fresh cilantro.
6. Adjust seasoning if needed and serve hot.

Nutrition: Calories: 250; Fat: 8g; Carbs: 35g; Protein: 10g; Sugar: 7g; Fiber: 9g;

Equipment: Large pot; Knife; Chopping board; Grater.

Sweet Potato and Black Bean Goulash

Prep time: 25 min　　**Total time:** 60 min
Cook time: 35 min　　**Servings:** 4

Ingredients:

- ✓ Sweet potatoes, peeled and diced, 3 cups
- ✓ Black beans, cooked, 2 cups
- ✓ Olive oil, 2 tbsp
- ✓ Red onion, thinly sliced, 1 cup
- ✓ Garlic cloves, minced, 3 pcs
- ✓ Celery, thinly sliced, 1 cup
- ✓ Cherry tomatoes, 1.5 cups
- ✓ Paprika, 2 tsp
- ✓ Black pepper, 1 pinch
- ✓ Salt, 1 pinch
- ✓ Water, 3 cups
- ✓ Fresh cilantro, chopped, 2 tbsp

Directions:

7. In a large pot, heat olive oil over medium heat. Add thinly sliced red onion and minced garlic, sauté until translucent.
8. Add the diced sweet potatoes and thinly sliced celery, continue sautéing for 5-7 minutes.
9. Mix in the cherry tomatoes, paprika, black pepper, and salt.
10. Pour in the black beans and water. Bring the mixture to a boil.
11. Once boiling, reduce the heat and let it simmer for 25-30 minutes, or until the sweet potatoes are tender.

12. Stir in the fresh cilantro just before serving. Adjust the seasoning if needed.

Nutrition: Calories: 270; Fat: 7g; Carbs: 45g; Protein: 9g; Sugar: 7g; Fiber: 10g;

Equipment: Large pot; Knife; Chopping board; Measuring cups and spoons.

Chicken and Green Bean Goulash

Prep time: 20 min   **Total time:** 50 min
Cook time: 30 min   **Servings:** 4

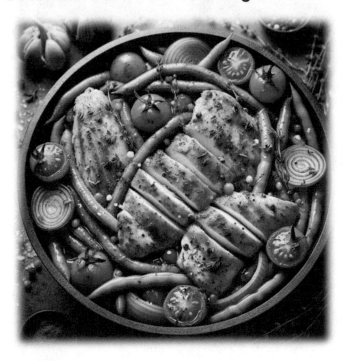

Ingredients:

✓ Grilled chicken breasts, sliced, 4 pcs
✓ Green beans, trimmed, 2 cups
✓ Olive oil, 2 tbsp
✓ Red onion, thinly sliced, 1 cup
✓ Garlic cloves, minced, 3 pcs
✓ Cherry tomatoes, 1.5 cups
✓ Paprika, 1 tsp
✓ Black pepper, 1 pinch
✓ Salt, 1 pinch
✓ Water, 2.5 cups
✓ Fresh thyme, chopped, 1 tbsp

Directions:

1. In a large pot, heat olive oil over medium heat. Add thinly sliced red onion and minced garlic, sauté until translucent.
2. Add the sliced grilled chicken breasts and sauté for 5 minutes.
3. Mix in the green beans, cherry tomatoes, paprika, black pepper, and salt.
4. Pour in the water. Bring the mixture to a boil.
5. Once boiling, reduce the heat and let it simmer for 20-25 minutes, or until the green beans are tender.
6. Stir in the chopped fresh thyme just before serving. Adjust the seasoning if needed.

Nutrition: Calories: 290; Fat: 10g; Carbs: 15g; Protein: 32g; Sugar: 6g; Fiber: 4g;

Equipment: Large pot; Knife; Chopping board; Measuring cups and spoons.

Shrimp and Broccoli Goulash in Lemon Herb Sauce

Prep time: 15 min   **Total time:** 40 min
Cook time: 25 min   **Servings:** 4

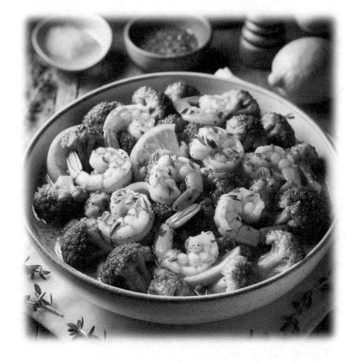

Ingredients:

- ✓ Shrimp, peeled and deveined, 1 lb
- ✓ Broccoli, cut into florets, 2 cups
- ✓ Olive oil, 2 tbsp
- ✓ Garlic cloves, minced, 3 pcs
- ✓ Fresh thyme, chopped, 1 tbsp
- ✓ Fresh dill, chopped, 1 tbsp
- ✓ Lemon zest, 1 lemon
- ✓ Black pepper, 1 pinch
- ✓ Salt, 1 pinch
- ✓ Water, 3 cups

Directions:

1. In a large pan, heat olive oil over medium heat. Add minced garlic and sauté until fragrant.
2. Add the shrimp and sauté for about 2-3 minutes until they start to turn pink.
3. Add the broccoli florets to the pan, mixing well.
4. Pour in the water and bring the mixture to a simmer.
5. Season with salt and black pepper.
6. Stir in the fresh thyme, fresh dill, and lemon zest.
7. Continue to simmer for 15-20 minutes until the broccoli is tender and the shrimp are fully cooked.
8. Adjust the seasoning if necessary before serving.

Nutrition: Calories: 210; Fat: 7g; Carbs: 10g; Protein: 25g; Sugar: 2g; Fiber: 3g;

Equipment: Large pan; Knife; Chopping board; Measuring cups and spoons; Zester.

Lentil and Swiss Chard Goulash

Prep time: 20 min **Total time:** 65 min
Cook time: 45 min **Servings:** 4

Ingredients:

- ✓ Dried green lentils, 1 cup
- ✓ Swiss chard, washed, stems removed and chopped, 4 cups
- ✓ Olive oil, 2 tbsp
- ✓ Garlic cloves, minced, 3 pcs
- ✓ Red onion, thinly sliced, 1 cup
- ✓ Black pepper, 1 pinch
- ✓ Salt, 1 pinch
- ✓ Water, 4 cups
- ✓ Paprika, 1 tsp
- ✓ Fresh thyme, chopped, 1 tbsp

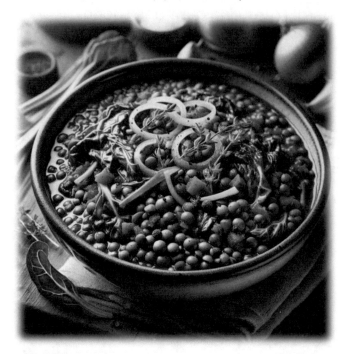

Directions:

1. Heat olive oil in a large pot over medium heat. Add the minced garlic and sliced red onion, sauté until translucent.
2. Add the dried green lentils to the pot, stirring well to coat them in the oil.
3. Sprinkle in the paprika, fresh thyme, salt, and black pepper. Mix well.
4. Pour in the water and bring the mixture to a boil.
5. Reduce the heat to low, cover, and simmer for 30 minutes, stirring occasionally.
6. Once the lentils are partially cooked, fold in the Swiss chard, allowing it to wilt in the heat of the goulash.
7. Continue cooking for another 10-15 minutes, or until the lentils are tender.
8. Adjust seasoning to taste and serve.

Nutrition: Calories: 260; Fat: 7g; Carbs: 38g; Protein: 14g; Sugar: 3g; Fiber: 10g;

Equipment: Large pot; Knife; Chopping board; Measuring cups and spoons.

Cod and Asparagus Goulash with Parsley

Prep time: 15 min   **Total time:** 45 min
Cook time: 30 min   **Servings:** 4

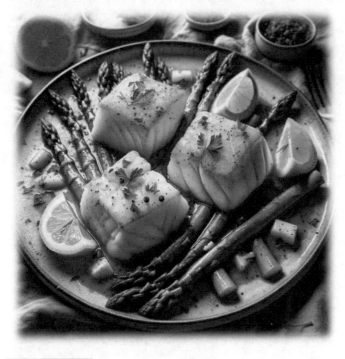

Ingredients:

- ✓ Cod fillets, 4 pcs (each about 6oz)
- ✓ Fresh asparagus, trimmed and cut into 2-inch pieces, 2 cups
- ✓ Olive oil, 2 tbsp
- ✓ Garlic cloves, minced, 3 pcs
- ✓ Black pepper, 1 pinch
- ✓ Salt, 1 pinch
- ✓ Water, 3 cups
- ✓ Chopped fresh parsley, 3 tbsp
- ✓ Paprika, 1 tsp
- ✓ Lemon zest, from 1 lemon
- ✓ Dijon mustard, 1 tsp

Directions:

1. Heat olive oil in a large skillet over medium heat. Add the minced garlic and sauté until fragrant.
2. Add the cod fillets to the skillet and sear each side for about 2 minutes or until slightly golden.
3. Sprinkle in the paprika, lemon zest, salt, and black pepper.
4. Pour in the water and bring to a gentle simmer.
5. Add the asparagus and cover the skillet. Let it simmer for about 15 minutes.
6. Mix in the Dijon mustard and cook for another 5 minutes, or until the cod is cooked through and the asparagus is tender.
7. Garnish with chopped fresh parsley and serve.

Nutrition: Calories: 210; Fat: 8g; Carbs: 5g; Protein: 30g; Sugar: 1g; Fiber: 2g;

Equipment: Large skillet; Knife; Chopping board; Measuring cups and spoons; Zester.

Lemon-Pepper Chicken Drumsticks

Prep time: 10 min   **Total time:** 55 min
Cook time: 45 min   **Servings:** 4

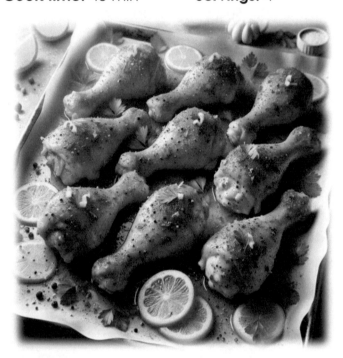

Ingredients:

✓ Chicken drumsticks, 8 pcs
✓ Olive oil, 2 tbsp
✓ Lemon zest, from 2 lemons
✓ Garlic cloves, minced, 3 pcs
✓ Black pepper, 2 pinches
✓ Salt, 1 pinch
✓ Chopped fresh parsley, 2 tbsp (for garnish)

Directions:

1. Preheat oven to 375°F (190°C).
2. In a large mixing bowl, combine olive oil, lemon zest, minced garlic, black pepper, and salt. Mix well.
3. Add the chicken drumsticks to the bowl and toss them until well coated with the mixture.
4. Arrange the drumsticks on a baking sheet lined with parchment paper.
5. Bake in the preheated oven for 40-45 minutes or until the chicken is golden brown and fully cooked.
6. Once cooked, remove from the oven and let them cool slightly.
7. Garnish with chopped fresh parsley before serving.

Nutrition: Calories: 280; Fat: 15g; Carbs: 1g; Protein: 34g; Sugar: 0g; Fiber: 0g;

Equipment: Large mixing bowl; Baking sheet; Parchment paper; Oven.

Grilled Turkey Patties with Lime and Cilantro

Prep time: 15 min   **Total time:** 30 min
Cook time: 15 min   **Servings:** 4

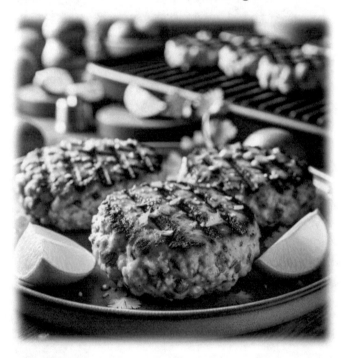

Ingredients:

✓ Ground turkey, 1 lb
✓ Fresh cilantro, chopped, 3 tbsp
✓ Lime zest, from 2 limes
✓ Garlic cloves, minced, 2 pcs
✓ Black pepper, 2 pinches
✓ Salt, 1 pinch
✓ Olive oil, for brushing, 1 tbsp

Directions:

1. In a large bowl, combine the ground turkey, chopped cilantro, lime zest, minced garlic, black pepper, and salt. Mix thoroughly.
2. Divide the mixture into 4 equal portions and shape each portion into a patty.
3. Preheat the grill to medium-high heat. Brush the grill grates with olive oil.
4. Place the patties on the grill and cook for about 6-7 minutes on each side, or until fully cooked and slightly charred.
5. Remove the patties from the grill and let them rest for a couple of minutes before serving.

Nutrition: Calories: 240; Fat: 14g; Carbs: 1g; Protein: 28g; Sugar: 0g; Fiber: 0g;

Equipment: Large bowl; Grill; Brush.

Spiced Beef Lettuce Wraps with Avocado

Prep time: 20 min
Cook time: 15 min

Total time: 35 min
Servings: 4

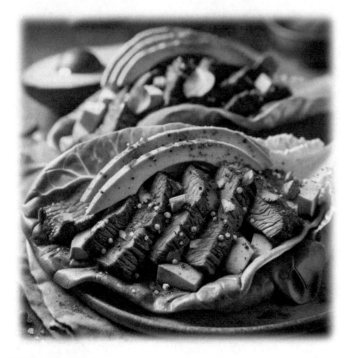

Ingredients:

✓ Beef strip steak, 16 oz

✓ Fresh spinach, 2 cups (to use as lettuce wraps)
✓ Avocado, sliced, 1 pcs
✓ Garlic cloves, minced, 2 pcs
✓ Olive oil, 2 tbsp
✓ Black pepper, 2 pinches
✓ Salt, 1 pinch
✓ Paprika, 1 tsp
✓ Lime zest, from 1 lime
✓ Fresh cilantro, chopped (for garnish), 2 tbsp

Directions:

1. Heat olive oil in a pan over medium-high heat.
2. Add the minced garlic and sauté for about 1 minute until fragrant.
3. Add the beef strip steak slices to the pan and cook until browned on both sides.
4. Season with salt, black pepper, paprika, and lime zest. Cook for another 2-3 minutes until the beef is fully cooked.
5. Remove from heat and let it rest for a couple of minutes.
6. Lay out fresh spinach leaves on plates. Place slices of beef on each spinach leaf.
7. Top with avocado slices and garnish with chopped cilantro.
8. Serve immediately and enjoy!

Nutrition: Calories: 320; Fat: 18g; Carbs: 9g; Protein: 32g; Sugar: 1g; Fiber: 5g;

Equipment: Pan; Knife; Serving plates.

Herb-Infused Chicken Skewers with Cherry Tomatoes

Prep time: 20 min
Cook time: 15 min

Total time: 35 min
Servings: 4

Ingredients:

✓ Chicken drumsticks, 8 pcs (skin removed and meat cut into cubes)
✓ Cherry tomatoes, 2 cups
✓ Olive oil, 2 tbsp
✓ Fresh thyme, chopped, 1 tbsp

- ✓ Fresh cilantro, chopped, 1 tbsp
- ✓ Garlic cloves, minced, 2 pcs
- ✓ Black pepper, 2 pinches
- ✓ Salt, 1 pinch
- ✓ Lemon zest, from 1 lemon

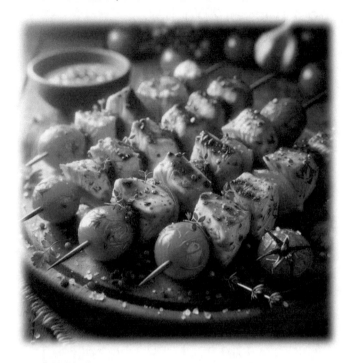

Directions:

1. In a large bowl, combine chicken cubes, olive oil, chopped thyme, chopped cilantro, minced garlic, black pepper, salt, and lemon zest. Mix well to ensure chicken is well coated.
2. Thread the chicken cubes and cherry tomatoes alternately onto skewers.
3. Preheat grill or grill pan over medium-high heat.
4. Place the skewers on the grill and cook for 5-7 minutes on each side, or until chicken is fully cooked and has grill marks.
5. Remove from grill and let them rest for a couple of minutes.
6. Serve hot with your favorite side dish or salad.

Nutrition: Calories: 210; Fat: 8g; Carbs: 7g; Protein: 28g; Sugar: 3g; Fiber: 1g;

Equipment: Grill or grill pan; Skewers; Large mixing bowl.

Honey-Mustard Glazed Pork Tenderloin

Prep time: 15 min   **Total time:** 40 min
Cook time: 25 min   **Servings:** 4

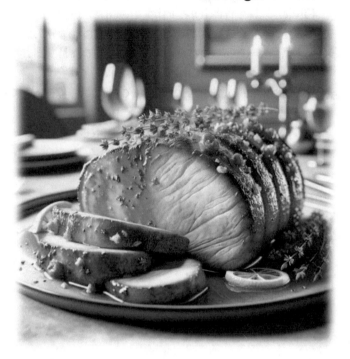

Ingredients:

- ✓ Pork tenderloin, 1 lb
- ✓ Honey, 3 tbsp
- ✓ Dijon mustard, 2 tsp
- ✓ Olive oil, 2 tbsp
- ✓ Garlic cloves, minced, 2 pcs
- ✓ Black pepper, 2 pinches
- ✓ Salt, 1 pinch
- ✓ Fresh thyme, chopped, 1 tbsp
- ✓ Lemon zest, from 1 lemon

Directions:

1. Preheat your oven to 375°F (190°C).
2. In a small bowl, combine honey, Dijon mustard, minced garlic, black pepper, salt, chopped thyme, and lemon zest. Mix well to create the glaze.
3. In a skillet or oven-proof pan, heat the olive oil over medium-high heat. Add the pork tenderloin and sear each side until golden brown, about 2-3 minutes per side.

4. Remove from heat and brush the tenderloin generously with the honey-mustard glaze.
5. Transfer the skillet or pan to the preheated oven and roast for 20-25 minutes or until the pork reaches an internal temperature of 145°F (63°C).
6. Once cooked, let the pork rest for 5 minutes before slicing. Serve with your preferred side dish.

Nutrition: Calories: 295; Fat: 11g; Carbs: 19g; Protein: 32g; Sugar: 17g; Fiber: 0.5g;

Equipment: Small bowl; Skillet or oven-proof pan; Oven; Brush or spoon for glazing.

Baked Turkey Sausage with Red Peppers and Onions

Prep time: 10 min   **Total time:** 45 min
Cook time: 35 min   **Servings:** 4

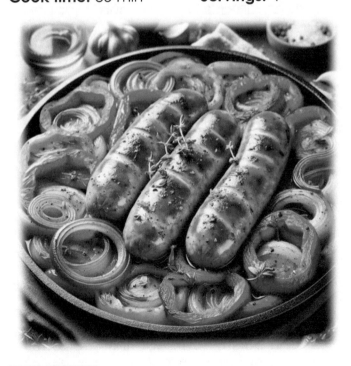

Ingredients:

✓ Turkey sausage, 1 lb
✓ Red bell peppers, sliced, 2 cups
✓ Red onion, thinly sliced, 1 cup
✓ Olive oil, 2 tbsp
✓ Black pepper, 2 pinches
✓ Salt, 1 pinch

✓ Fresh thyme, chopped, 1 tbsp
✓ Garlic cloves, minced, 2 pcs

Directions:

1. Preheat the oven to 400°F (205°C).
2. In a large mixing bowl, combine sliced red bell peppers, thinly sliced red onion, minced garlic, chopped thyme, olive oil, salt, and black pepper. Toss to coat.
3. Lay the turkey sausages in a baking dish and surround them with the pepper and onion mixture.
4. Place the baking dish in the oven and bake for 30-35 minutes or until the sausages are cooked through and the vegetables are tender.
5. Remove from the oven and let cool for a few minutes before serving.

Nutrition: Calories: 320; Fat: 17g; Carbs: 10g; Protein: 28g; Sugar: 4g; Fiber: 2g;

Equipment: Oven; Large mixing bowl; Baking dish.

Rosemary Beef Tips with Brussels Sprouts

Prep time: 15 min   **Total time:** 40 min
Cook time: 25 min   **Servings:** 4

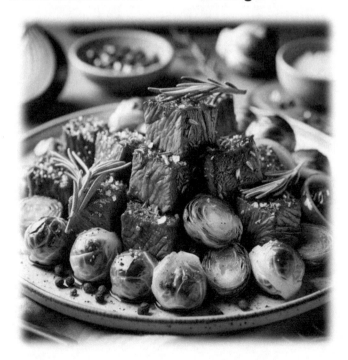

Ingredients:

- ✓ Beef strip steak, cubed, 16 oz
- ✓ Brussels sprouts, halved, 2 cups
- ✓ Olive oil, 3 tbsp
- ✓ Fresh rosemary, finely chopped, 2 tbsp
- ✓ Garlic cloves, minced, 3 pcs
- ✓ Black pepper, 2 pinches
- ✓ Salt, 1 pinch
- ✓ Red onion, thinly sliced, 1/2 cup

Directions:

1. Preheat the oven to 400°F (205°C).
2. In a large mixing bowl, toss the Brussels sprouts with 1 tablespoon of olive oil, a pinch of salt, and a pinch of black pepper. Spread them on a baking sheet in a single layer and roast in the oven for 20 minutes or until they are golden and tender.
3. Meanwhile, in a large skillet, heat 2 tablespoons of olive oil over medium-high heat. Add the red onion slices and sauté for 2-3 minutes until they begin to soften.
4. Add the beef cubes to the skillet. Season with rosemary, minced garlic, salt, and black pepper. Cook until the beef is browned on all sides, about 7-8 minutes.
5. Once the Brussels sprouts are done roasting, add them to the skillet with the beef, and toss everything together to combine. Cook for another 2-3 minutes, then serve immediately.

Nutrition: Calories: 340; Fat: 18g; Carbs: 12g; Protein: 32g; Sugar: 3g; Fiber: 4g;

Equipment: Oven; Large mixing bowl; Baking sheet; Large skillet.

Stuffed Chicken Thighs with Quinoa and Asparagus

Prep time: 20 min   **Total time:** 60 min
Cook time: 40 min   **Servings:** 4

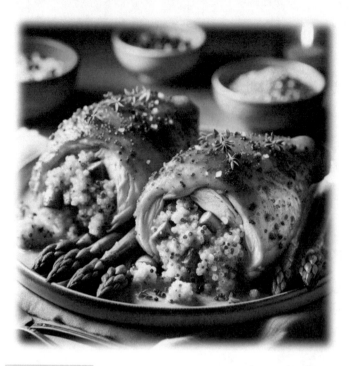

Ingredients:

- ✓ Chicken drumsticks, boneless and skinless, 8 pcs
- ✓ Quinoa, 1 cup
- ✓ Fresh asparagus, trimmed and chopped, 1 cup
- ✓ Olive oil, 2 tbsp
- ✓ Garlic cloves, minced, 2 pcs
- ✓ Salt, 1 pinch
- ✓ Black pepper, 2 pinches
- ✓ Fresh thyme, chopped, 1 tbsp
- ✓ Water, 2 cups

Directions:

1. Preheat the oven to 375°F (190°C).
2. In a medium-sized pot, bring water to a boil. Add the quinoa, cover, and reduce heat to low. Cook for about 15 minutes or until quinoa is fluffy and all the water is absorbed. Let it cool.
3. In a skillet, heat 1 tablespoon of olive oil over medium heat. Add the chopped asparagus and sauté for 4-5 minutes or until tender. Add the minced garlic and sauté for another minute. Mix this with the cooked quinoa, then season with salt, black pepper, and fresh thyme.
4. Carefully stuff each chicken drumstick with the quinoa and asparagus mixture.

5. In a large ovenproof skillet, heat the remaining tablespoon of olive oil over medium-high heat. Add the stuffed chicken drumsticks and brown on all sides, about 4-5 minutes.
6. Transfer the skillet to the preheated oven and bake for about 25-30 minutes or until chicken is fully cooked.
7. Serve hot and enjoy!

Nutrition: Calories: 380; Fat: 14g; Carbs: 35g; Protein: 28g; Sugar: 1g; Fiber: 5g;

Equipment: Oven; Medium-sized pot; Skillet; Mixing bowl.

Lamb Meatballs with Mint and Lemon Zest

Prep time: 15 min
Cook time: 25 min

Total time: 40 min
Servings: 4

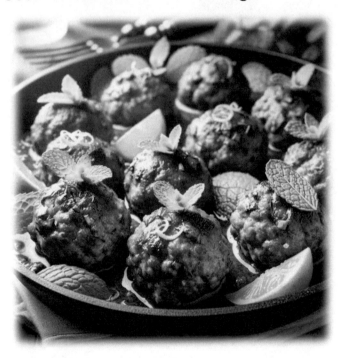

Ingredients:

✓ Ground lamb, 1 lb
✓ Fresh mint leaves, finely chopped, 20 leaves
✓ Lemon zest from 1 lemon
✓ Eggs, 1 pc
✓ Garlic cloves, minced, 2 pcs
✓ Salt, 1 pinch

✓ Black pepper, 1 pinch
✓ Olive oil, 2 tbsp

Directions:

1. In a large mixing bowl, combine the ground lamb, chopped mint leaves, lemon zest, minced garlic, and egg. Mix until well combined.
2. Season the mixture with salt and black pepper. Mix again.
3. Shape the mixture into small meatballs, about the size of a golf ball.
4. Heat olive oil in a large skillet over medium-high heat.
5. Place the meatballs in the skillet and brown on all sides, about 5-7 minutes.
6. Reduce heat to medium, cover, and cook for an additional 15-18 minutes, turning occasionally, until meatballs are cooked through.
7. Serve hot and enjoy!

Nutrition: Calories: 330; Fat: 24g; Carbs: 2g; Protein: 23g; Sugar: 0g; Fiber: 0.5g;

Equipment: Large mixing bowl; Skillet; Mixing spoon.

Pomegranate-Glazed Chicken Wings

Prep time: 15 min
Cook time: 40 min

Total time: 55 min
Servings: 4

Ingredients:

✓ Chicken drumsticks, 12 pcs
✓ Fresh mint leaves, finely chopped, 15 leaves
✓ Honey, 3 tbsp
✓ Olive oil, 2 tbsp
✓ Pomegranate juice, 1 cup
✓ Garlic cloves, minced, 3 pcs
✓ Salt, 1 pinch
✓ Black pepper, 1 pinch

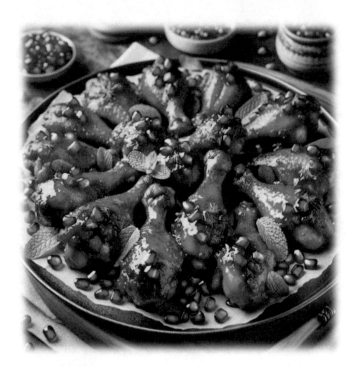

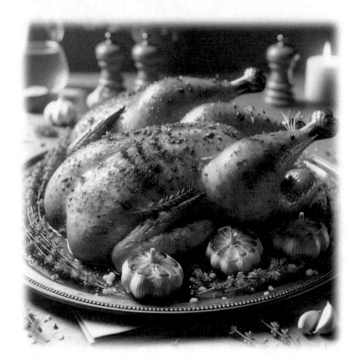

Directions:

1. Preheat your oven to 375°F (190°C).
2. In a large bowl, whisk together the pomegranate juice, honey, olive oil, minced garlic, salt, and black pepper until well combined.
3. Toss the chicken drumsticks in the mixture until they're well coated.
4. Place the coated chicken drumsticks on a baking sheet lined with parchment paper.
5. Bake in the preheated oven for 35-40 minutes or until the chicken is fully cooked and the glaze has caramelized.
6. Remove from the oven and let cool for a few minutes.
7. Sprinkle the finely chopped mint leaves over the top before serving.

Nutrition: Calories: 310; Fat: 14g; Carbs: 18g; Protein: 28g; Sugar: 14g; Fiber: 0.5g;

Equipment: Large bowl; Baking sheet; Parchment paper; Whisk.

Garlic Butter Roasted Cornish Hen

Prep time: 20 min   **Total time:** 70 min
Cook time: 50 min   **Servings:** 2

Ingredients:

✓ Cornish hens, 2 pcs
✓ Garlic cloves, minced, 4 pcs
✓ Olive oil, 3 tbsp
✓ Fresh rosemary, finely chopped, 2 tbsp
✓ Fresh thyme, chopped, 1 tbsp
✓ Salt, 1 pinch
✓ Black pepper, 1 pinch
✓ Lemon zest, 1 lemon

Directions:

1. Preheat your oven to 375°F (190°C).
2. In a bowl, combine the minced garlic, olive oil, chopped rosemary, chopped thyme, lemon zest, salt, and black pepper. Mix well.
3. Clean the Cornish hens and pat them dry. Rub the garlic butter mixture all over the hens, both inside and outside.
4. Place the hens on a roasting tray, breast side up.
5. Roast in the preheated oven for 50 minutes, or until the internal temperature reaches 165°F (74°C) and the skin is golden brown.
6. Let the hens rest for about 10 minutes before serving.

Nutrition: Calories: 480; Fat: 34g; Carbs: 5g; Protein: 38g; Sugar: 1g; Fiber: 0.5g;

Equipment: Oven; Bowl; Roasting tray; Meat thermometer.

Beef and Mushroom Stir-Fry with Broccoli

Prep time: 15 min
Cook time: 10 min

Total time: 25 min
Servings: 4

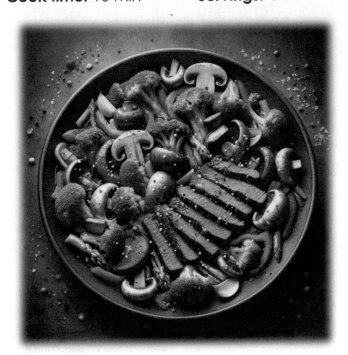

Ingredients:

✓ Beef strip steak, 16 oz, thinly sliced
✓ Portobello mushrooms, 4 large caps, sliced
✓ Broccoli, 2 cups, cut into small florets
✓ Garlic cloves, minced, 3 pcs
✓ Olive oil, 2 tbsp
✓ Soy sauce (low sodium), 2 tbsp
✓ Honey, 1 tbsp
✓ Red bell peppers, sliced, 1 cup
✓ Black pepper, 1 pinch
✓ Salt, 1 pinch

Directions:

1. In a mixing bowl, combine soy sauce, honey, minced garlic, salt, and black pepper. Mix well.
2. Add the thinly sliced beef to the mixture and let it marinate for about 10 minutes.
3. Heat olive oil in a large skillet or wok over medium-high heat.

4. Add the beef to the skillet and stir-fry for about 3-4 minutes until it's almost cooked through.
5. Add the sliced mushrooms, broccoli florets, and red bell peppers. Continue to stir-fry for another 5 minutes, or until the vegetables are tender and the beef is fully cooked.
6. Serve immediately.

Nutrition: Calories: 290; Fat: 10g; Carbs: 20g; Protein: 30g; Sugar: 8g; Fiber: 4g;

Equipment: Large skillet or wok; Mixing bowl.

Cilantro-Lime Chicken with Avocado Salsa

Prep time: 20 min
Cook time: 15 min

Total time: 35 min
Servings: 4

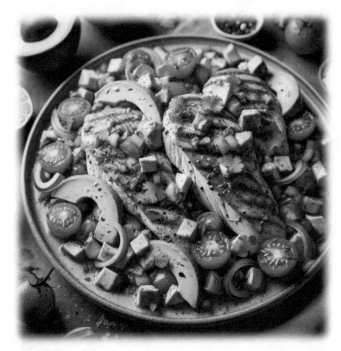

Ingredients:

✓ Grilled chicken breasts, 4 pcs
✓ Fresh cilantro, chopped, 3 tbsp
✓ Lime zest, 1 lime
✓ Avocado, 2 pcs, diced
✓ Cherry tomatoes, 1 cup, halved
✓ Red onion, thinly sliced, 1/2 cup
✓ Olive oil, 2 tbsp
✓ Black pepper, 1 pinch

✓ Salt, 1 pinch
✓ Garlic cloves, minced, 2 pcs

Directions:

7. In a small bowl, mix together olive oil, fresh cilantro, lime zest, minced garlic, salt, and black pepper.
8. Marinate the chicken breasts in the mixture for at least 15 minutes.
9. Grill the chicken breasts over medium-high heat for 6-7 minutes on each side or until cooked through.
10. In another bowl, combine diced avocado, halved cherry tomatoes, and thinly sliced red onion.
11. Serve the grilled chicken topped with the avocado salsa. Drizzle with additional lime juice if desired.

Nutrition: Calories: 320; Fat: 15g; Carbs: 12g; Protein: 35g; Sugar: 3g; Fiber: 7g;

Equipment: Grill; Mixing bowls.

Smoked Paprika Pork Ribs with Roasted Vegetable Medley

Prep time: 25 min   **Total time:** 175 min
Cook time: 150 min   **Servings:** 4

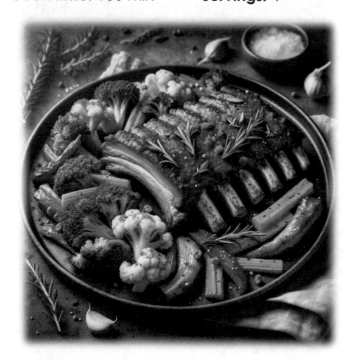

Ingredients:

✓ Pork ribs, 2 lb (not mentioned in the table but essential for the recipe)
✓ Paprika, 2 tsp
✓ Olive oil, 2 tbsp
✓ Salt, 1 pinch
✓ Black pepper, 1 pinch
✓ Broccoli, 2 cups, cut into florets
✓ Cauliflower, 2 cups, cut into florets
✓ Carrot, chopped, 2 cups
✓ Red bell peppers, sliced, 1 cup
✓ Garlic cloves, minced, 3 pcs
✓ Fresh rosemary, finely chopped, 1 tbsp
✓ Fresh thyme, chopped, 1 tbsp

Directions:

1. Preheat oven to 275°F (135°C).
2. In a small bowl, combine paprika, 1 tbsp olive oil, salt, and black pepper to make a rub. Spread the rub evenly over the pork ribs.
3. Place the ribs in the oven and bake for about 2 hours.
4. While the ribs are baking, in a large mixing bowl, combine broccoli, cauliflower, grated carrot, sliced red bell peppers, minced garlic, fresh rosemary, fresh thyme, 1 tbsp olive oil, salt, and black pepper. Toss until vegetables are well-coated.
5. Once the ribs have baked for 2 hours, increase the oven temperature to 400°F (205°C).
6. Spread the vegetable mixture on a baking sheet and place in the oven. Roast the vegetables for 30 minutes or until tender and slightly browned.
7. Serve the pork ribs alongside the roasted vegetable medley.

Nutrition: Calories: 500; Fat: 35g; Carbs: 25g; Protein: 45g; Sugar: 7g; Fiber: 8g;

Equipment: Oven; Mixing bowls; Baking sheet.

FISH RECIPES

Lemon-Pepper Baked Mackerel

Prep time: 10 min
Cook time: 25 min

Total time: 35 min
Servings: 4

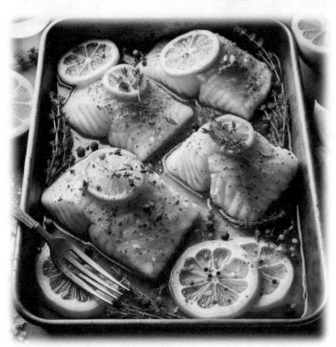

Ingredients:

- ✓ Fresh mackerel fillets, 4 pcs
- ✓ Olive oil, 2 tbsp
- ✓ Lemon zest, 2 lemons
- ✓ Black pepper, 2 pinches
- ✓ Salt, 1 pinch
- ✓ Garlic cloves, minced, 3 pcs
- ✓ Fresh thyme, chopped, 1 tbsp
- ✓ Fresh rosemary, finely chopped, 1 tbsp

Directions:

1. Preheat the oven to 375°F (190°C).
2. In a bowl, mix olive oil, lemon zest, minced garlic, black pepper, salt, chopped thyme, and finely chopped rosemary to form a marinade.
3. Place the mackerel fillets on a baking dish and coat them with the marinade.

4. Bake in the oven for about 20-25 minutes or until the mackerel is cooked through and easily flakes with a fork.
5. Once cooked, remove from the oven and serve hot. Garnish with additional lemon zest or herbs if desired.

Nutrition: Calories: 300; Fat: 20g; Carbs: 2g; Protein: 25g; Sugar: 0g; Fiber: 1g;

Equipment: Oven; Mixing bowl; Baking dish.

Tilapia with Tomato-Basil Relish

Prep time: 15 min
Cook time: 10 min

Total time: 25 min
Servings: 4

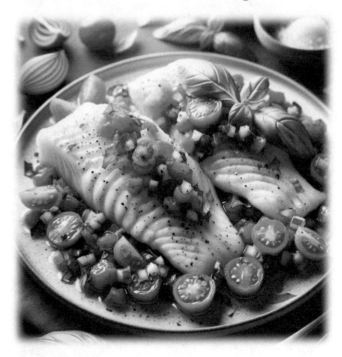

Ingredients:

- ✓ Tilapia fillets, 4 oz each, 4 pcs
- ✓ Olive oil, 2 tbsp
- ✓ Salt, 1 pinch
- ✓ Black pepper, 1 pinch
- ✓ Cherry tomatoes, quartered, 2 cups
- ✓ Fresh basil leaves, finely chopped, 10 leaves
- ✓ Red onion, thinly sliced, 1/2 cup
- ✓ Garlic cloves, minced, 2 pcs
- ✓ White wine vinegar, 1 tbsp
- ✓ Lemon zest, 1 lemon

Directions:

1. Preheat a grill or grill pan over medium heat.
2. Season the tilapia fillets with salt, black pepper, and 1 tbsp of olive oil.
3. Grill the tilapia for 4-5 minutes on each side or until cooked through and flaky.
4. In a mixing bowl, combine cherry tomatoes, fresh basil, red onion, minced garlic, white wine vinegar, the remaining olive oil, and lemon zest. Toss well to combine.
5. Serve the grilled tilapia on plates and top with the tomato-basil relish.

Nutrition: Calories: 240; Fat: 10g; Carbs: 5g; Protein: 30g; Sugar: 3g; Fiber: 1g;

Equipment: Grill or grill pan; Mixing bowl; Knife.

Garlic and Herb Crusted Whitefish (Cod)

Prep time: 15 min
Cook time: 20 min
Total time: 35 min
Servings: 4

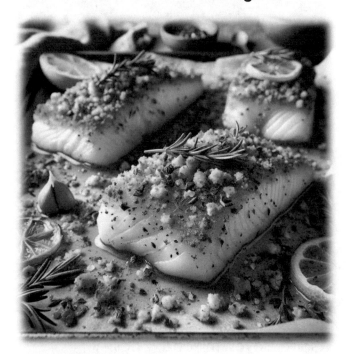

Ingredients:

✓ Cod fillets, 4 oz each, 4 pcs
✓ Olive oil, 2 tbsp
✓ Salt, 1 pinch
✓ Black pepper, 1 pinch
✓ Garlic cloves, minced, 4 pcs
✓ Fresh rosemary, finely chopped, 1 tbsp
✓ Fresh thyme, chopped, 1 tbsp
✓ Lemon zest, 1 lemon
✓ Whole grain bread, 2 slices, crushed into breadcrumbs

Directions:

1. Preheat oven to 400°F (205°C).
2. Lay the cod fillets on a baking sheet lined with parchment paper.
3. In a small bowl, combine olive oil, minced garlic, chopped rosemary, chopped thyme, and lemon zest to form a paste.
4. Season the cod fillets with salt and black pepper.
5. Spread the garlic and herb mixture evenly over each cod fillet.
6. Sprinkle crushed whole grain breadcrumbs on top of each fillet, pressing lightly to adhere.
7. Bake in the oven for 15-20 minutes or until the fish flakes easily with a fork and the crust is golden brown.

Nutrition: Calories: 220; Fat: 8g; Carbs: 10g; Protein: 30g; Sugar: 1g; Fiber: 2g;

Equipment: Oven; Baking sheet; Parchment paper; Mixing bowl; Knife.

Simple Shrimp and Broccoli Stir-Fry

Prep time: 10 min
Cook time: 10 min
Total time: 20 min
Servings: 4

Ingredients:

✓ Shrimp, peeled and deveined, 1 lb
✓ Broccoli, 2 cups
✓ Olive oil, 2 tbsp
✓ Garlic cloves, minced, 3 pcs
✓ Soy sauce (low sodium), 2 tbsp
✓ Black pepper, 1 pinch

- ✓ Water, 1/4 cup
- ✓ Red bell peppers, sliced, 1 cup
- ✓ Salt, 1 pinch

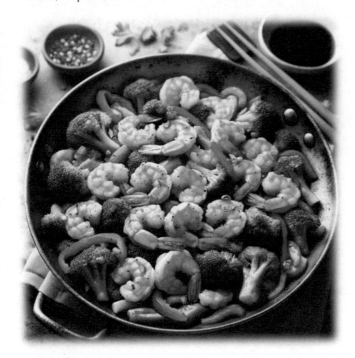

Directions:

1. Heat olive oil in a large skillet or wok over medium-high heat.
2. Add minced garlic and stir-fry for about 1 minute until fragrant.
3. Add shrimp to the skillet and cook until pink, about 2-3 minutes per side.
4. Remove the shrimp and set aside.
5. In the same skillet, add broccoli and sliced red bell peppers, stir-frying for about 4 minutes.
6. Add water to the skillet and cover, letting the broccoli steam until tender, about 3-4 minutes.
7. Return the shrimp to the skillet. Add low sodium soy sauce, salt, and black pepper, and stir-fry for another 2 minutes, ensuring all ingredients are well combined and heated through.

Nutrition: Calories: 210; Fat: 7g; Carbs: 9g; Protein: 28g; Sugar: 3g; Fiber: 3g;

Equipment: Large skillet or wok; Wooden spatula; Knife; Cutting board.

Pan-Fried Catfish with Lemon Aioli

Prep time: 15 min   **Total time:** 25 min
Cook time: 10 min   **Servings:** 4

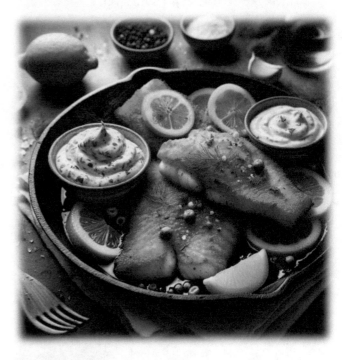

Ingredients:

- ✓ Catfish fillets, 4 pcs (approximately 6 oz each)
- ✓ Olive oil, 3 tbsp
- ✓ All-purpose flour, 1/2 cup
- ✓ Salt, 1 pinch
- ✓ Black pepper, 1 pinch
- ✓ Garlic cloves, minced, 2 pcs
- ✓ Greek yogurt, 1/2 cup
- ✓ Lemon zest, 1 lemon
- ✓ Fresh dill, chopped, 1 tbsp

Directions:

1. In a shallow dish, combine all-purpose flour, salt, and black pepper.
2. Dredge each catfish fillet in the flour mixture, shaking off the excess.
3. Heat 2 tbsp of olive oil in a large skillet over medium-high heat.
4. Add catfish fillets and pan-fry for 4-5 minutes on each side, or until golden brown and cooked through.
5. In a small mixing bowl, combine minced garlic, Greek yogurt, 1 tbsp of olive oil, lemon zest, and fresh dill to make the lemon aioli.

6. Serve catfish fillets hot with a dollop of lemon aioli on the side.

Nutrition: Calories: 310; Fat: 14g; Carbs: 12g; Protein: 34g; Sugar: 2g; Fiber: 1g;

Equipment: Large skillet; Mixing bowl; Shallow dish; Spoon.

Spiced Cod with Fresh Tomato Salsa

Prep time: 20 min   **Total time:** 30 min
Cook time: 10 min   **Servings:** 4

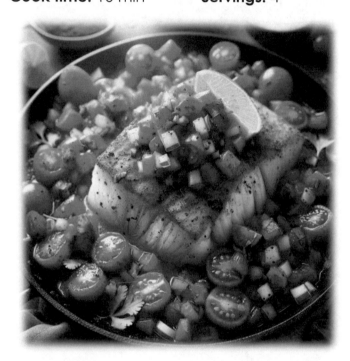

Ingredients:

✓ Cod fillets, 4 pcs (approximately 6 oz each)
✓ Olive oil, 2 tbsp
✓ Paprika, 1 tsp
✓ Black pepper, 1 pinch
✓ Salt, 1 pinch
✓ Cherry tomatoes, 2 cups, finely diced and halved
✓ Red onion, thinly sliced, 1/2 cup
✓ Fresh cilantro, chopped, 2 tbsp
✓ Lime zest, 1 lime
✓ Garlic cloves, minced, 2 pcs

Directions:

1. In a bowl, combine the paprika, black pepper, and salt. Rub the spice mixture onto both sides of each cod fillet.
2. Heat 1 tbsp of olive oil in a skillet over medium heat. Add the cod fillets and cook for about 4-5 minutes on each side, or until the fish flakes easily with a fork.
3. In a separate bowl, combine the cherry tomatoes, red onion, fresh cilantro, lime zest, minced garlic, and remaining olive oil to make the fresh tomato salsa. Mix well.
4. Serve the spiced cod fillets hot and top with a generous portion of fresh tomato salsa.

Nutrition: Calories: 220; Fat: 8g; Carbs: 6g; Protein: 30g; Sugar: 3g; Fiber: 2g;

Equipment: Mixing bowl; Skillet; Spoon.

Shrimp and Corn Quesadillas

Prep time: 15 min   **Total time:** 30 min
Cook time: 15 min   **Servings:** 4

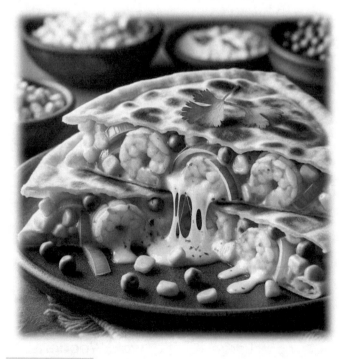

Ingredients:

✓ Shrimp, peeled and deveined, 1 lb
✓ Olive oil, 2 tbsp

- ✓ Red onion, thinly sliced, 1/2 cup
- ✓ Green peas, 1 cup
- ✓ Mozzarella cheese, 2 cups
- ✓ Whole wheat pita pockets, 4 pcs
- ✓ Black pepper, 1 pinch
- ✓ Salt, 1 pinch
- ✓ Garlic cloves, minced, 2 pcs
- ✓ Fresh cilantro, chopped, 2 tbsp

Directions:

1. In a skillet over medium heat, add 1 tbsp of olive oil. Add minced garlic and sauté until fragrant.
2. Add the shrimp and cook until they turn pink, about 2-3 minutes on each side. Remove from skillet and set aside.
3. In the same skillet, add the thinly sliced red onion and green peas. Sauté until the onions become translucent.
4. Return the whole cooked shrimp to the skillet. Season with salt and black pepper.
5. On a separate pan, place one pita pocket. Add a layer of mozzarella cheese, then the shrimp and vegetable mixture, followed by another layer of cheese. Top with another pita pocket.
6. Cook on each side until the pita is golden brown and the cheese has melted.
7. Remove from heat, sprinkle with fresh cilantro, and serve hot.

Nutrition: Calories: 320; Fat: 12g; Carbs: 25g; Protein: 28g; Sugar: 3g; Fiber: 4g;

Equipment: Skillet; Cooking spatula.

Baked Trout with Orange and Rosemary

Prep time: 10 min **Total time:** 30 min
Cook time: 20 min **Servings:** 4

Ingredients:

- ✓ Fresh trout fillets, 4 oz each
- ✓ Orange, zested and juiced, 1 pc
- ✓ Fresh rosemary, finely chopped, 1 tbsp

- ✓ Olive oil, 2 tbsp
- ✓ Garlic cloves, minced, 2 pcs
- ✓ Salt, 1 pinch
- ✓ Black pepper, 1 pinch

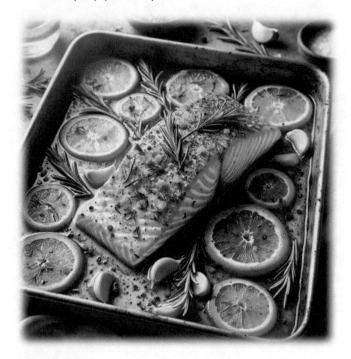

Directions:

1. Preheat oven to 400°F (200°C).
2. In a bowl, combine olive oil, minced garlic, orange zest, orange juice, and chopped rosemary. Mix well.
3. Place the trout fillets in a baking dish, skin side down.
4. Drizzle the orange and rosemary mixture over the trout.
5. Season with a pinch of salt and black pepper.
6. Bake in the preheated oven for 15-20 minutes or until the trout flakes easily with a fork.
7. Remove from oven and serve immediately.

Nutrition: Calories: 200; Fat: 9g; Carbs: 4g; Protein: 26g; Sugar: 2g; Fiber: 0.5g;

Equipment: Oven; Baking dish; Mixing bowl.

Ginger-Soy Glazed Haddock

Prep time: 15 min   **Total time:** 30 min
Cook time: 15 min   **Servings:** 4

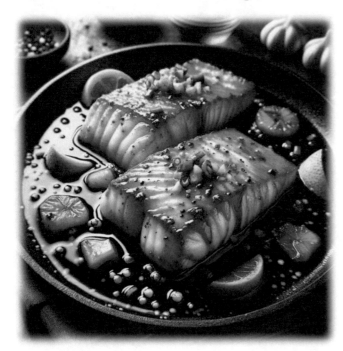

Ingredients:

- ✓ Haddock fillets, 4 oz each
- ✓ Soy sauce (low sodium), 3 tbsp
- ✓ Honey, 2 tbsp
- ✓ Garlic cloves, minced, 2 pcs
- ✓ Fresh ginger, grated, 1 tbsp
- ✓ Olive oil, 1 tbsp
- ✓ Black pepper, 1 pinch

Directions:

1. In a mixing bowl, combine soy sauce, honey, minced garlic, and grated ginger. Stir well until honey is dissolved.
2. Place the haddock fillets in a shallow dish and pour the ginger-soy mixture over them. Marinate for 10 minutes.
3. Heat olive oil in a skillet over medium-high heat. Remove haddock from the marinade, reserving the liquid, and place in the skillet.
4. Cook haddock for about 3-4 minutes on each side or until opaque.
5. Pour the reserved marinade into the skillet and let it simmer until it reduces to a glaze.

6. Spoon the glaze over the haddock and serve immediately.

Nutrition: Calories: 220; Fat: 6g; Carbs: 10g; Protein: 30g; Sugar: 9g; Fiber: 0g;

Equipment: Mixing bowl; Shallow dish; Skillet.

Flounder Fillets with Cilantro and Lime

Prep time: 10 min   **Total time:** 25 min
Cook time: 15 min   **Servings:** 4

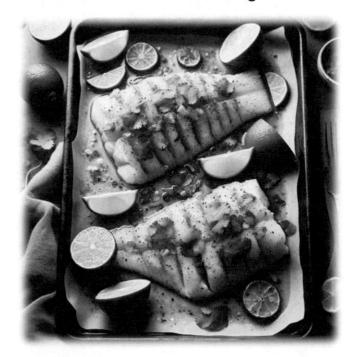

Ingredients:

- ✓ Flounder fillets, 4 oz each
- ✓ Lime zest, 1 lime
- ✓ Fresh cilantro, chopped, 3 tbsp
- ✓ Olive oil, 2 tbsp
- ✓ Black pepper, 1 pinch
- ✓ Salt, 1 pinch

Directions:

1. Preheat your oven to 375°F (190°C).
2. In a small bowl, mix together lime zest, chopped cilantro, salt, and pepper.
3. Place flounder fillets on a baking sheet lined with parchment paper.
4. Brush each fillet with olive oil.

5. Sprinkle the cilantro and lime mixture evenly over each fillet.
6. Bake in the preheated oven for 10-12 minutes or until flounder is opaque and flakes easily with a fork.

Nutrition: Calories: 180; Fat: 8g; Carbs: 2g; Protein: 25g; Sugar: 0g; Fiber: 0g;

Equipment: Oven; Small bowl; Baking sheet; Parchment paper.

Shrimp Tacos with Cabbage Slaw

Prep time: 15 min   **Total time:** 25 min
Cook time: 10 min   **Servings:** 4

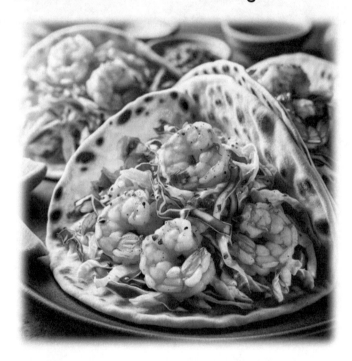

Ingredients:

✓ Shrimp, peeled and deveined, 1 lb
✓ Green cabbage, 2 cups
✓ Red onion, thinly sliced, 1 cup
✓ Fresh cilantro, chopped, 2 tbsp
✓ Olive oil, 2 tbsp
✓ Lime zest, 1 lime
✓ Soy sauce (low sodium), 1 tbsp
✓ Black pepper, 1 pinch
✓ Salt, 1 pinch
✓ Whole wheat pita pockets, 4 pcs

Directions:

1. In a large bowl, combine the green cabbage, red onion, and fresh cilantro. Mix well.
2. In a separate bowl, whisk together olive oil, lime zest, soy sauce, black pepper, and salt. Pour this dressing over the cabbage slaw and toss to coat evenly.
3. In a skillet over medium heat, add a tablespoon of olive oil. Once hot, add the shrimp and cook for 2-3 minutes on each side or until they turn pink and are fully cooked.
4. Warm the whole wheat pita pockets in the oven or on a skillet.
5. Assemble the tacos by adding the shrimp to each pita pocket and topping with the cabbage slaw.

Nutrition: Calories: 350; Fat: 12g; Carbs: 30g; Protein: 30g; Sugar: 4g; Fiber: 5g;

Equipment: Large bowl; Skillet; Small bowl.

Baked Salmon Patties with Dill Sauce

Prep time: 20 min   **Total time:** 45 min
Cook time: 25 min   **Servings:** 4

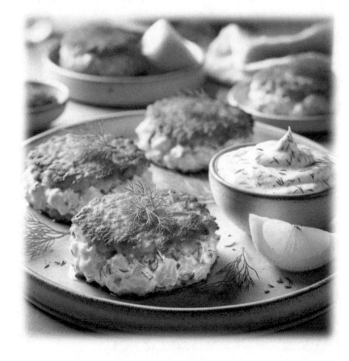

Ingredients:

- ✓ Smoked salmon, 8 oz
- ✓ Whole grain bread, 2 slices (crumbled)
- ✓ Eggs, 2 pcs
- ✓ Fresh dill, chopped, 2 tbsp
- ✓ Red onion, thinly sliced, 1/2 cup
- ✓ Greek yogurt, 1/2 cup
- ✓ Dijon mustard, 1 tsp
- ✓ Lemon zest, 1 lemon
- ✓ Olive oil, 1 tbsp
- ✓ Black pepper, 1 pinch
- ✓ Salt, 1 pinch

Directions:

1. Preheat the oven to 375°F (190°C).
2. In a bowl, combine the smoked salmon, crumbled whole grain bread, 1 egg, 1 tbsp of fresh dill, and half of the sliced red onion. Mix well.
3. Form the mixture into 4 patties and place on a baking sheet lined with parchment paper.
4. Drizzle the patties with olive oil and bake for 20-25 minutes or until golden and firm.
5. While the patties are baking, prepare the dill sauce. In a bowl, combine the Greek yogurt, Dijon mustard, 1 tbsp of fresh dill, lemon zest, and remaining egg. Whisk until smooth.
6. Once the patties are done, serve with the dill sauce on the side.

Nutrition: Calories: 210; Fat: 8g; Carbs: 10g; Protein: 25g; Sugar: 3g; Fiber: 2g;

Equipment: Oven; Mixing bowl; Baking sheet; Parchment paper; Whisk.

Grilled Red Snapper with Avocado and Mango Relish

Prep time: 15 min   **Total time:** 25 min
Cook time: 10 min   **Servings:** 4

Ingredients:

- ✓ Red snapper fillets, 4 (each approx. 6 oz)
- ✓ Avocado, thinly sliced, 2 pcs
- ✓ Fresh mango, 2 pcs (diced)
- ✓ Red onion, thinly sliced, 1/2 cup
- ✓ Fresh cilantro, chopped, 2 tbsp
- ✓ Olive oil, 2 tbsp
- ✓ Lime zest, 1 lime
- ✓ Salt, 1 pinch
- ✓ Black pepper, 1 pinch

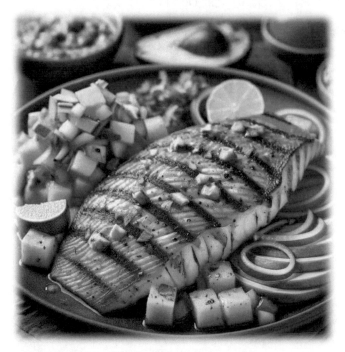

Directions:

1. Preheat the grill to medium-high heat.
2. In a medium-sized bowl, combine the diced avocado, diced mango, thinly sliced red onion, chopped cilantro, and lime zest. Mix well and set aside.
3. Brush the red snapper fillets with 1 tbsp olive oil on both sides and season with salt and black pepper.
4. Grill the red snapper fillets for about 4-5 minutes on each side or until fully cooked through.
5. Serve the grilled red snapper fillets with the avocado and mango relish on the side.

Nutrition: Calories: 270; Fat: 12g; Carbs: 20g; Protein: 25g; Sugar: 10g; Fiber: 5g;

Equipment: Grill: Medium-sized bowl; Brush.

Herb-Buttered Sea Bass with Asparagus

Prep time: 10 min   **Total time:** 25 min
Cook time: 15 min   **Servings:** 4

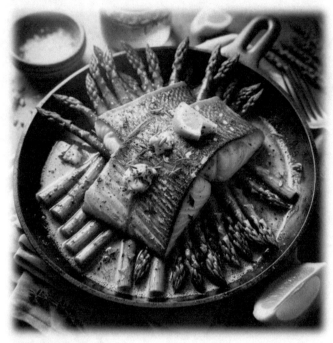

Ingredients:

✓ Sea bass fillets, 4 (each approx. 6 oz)
✓ Fresh asparagus, 2 cups (trimmed)
✓ Olive oil, 2 tbsp
✓ Fresh rosemary, finely chopped, 1 tbsp
✓ Fresh thyme, chopped, 1 tbsp
✓ Garlic cloves, minced, 2 pcs
✓ Salt, 1 pinch
✓ Black pepper, 1 pinch
✓ Lemon zest, 1 lemon
✓ Butter, 2 tbsp (unsalted)

Directions:

1. In a small bowl, combine the butter, finely chopped rosemary, chopped thyme, minced garlic, and lemon zest. Mix until well combined.
2. Preheat a skillet over medium-high heat. Add 1 tbsp olive oil.
3. Season the sea bass fillets with salt and black pepper. Add them to the skillet and cook for about 3-4 minutes on each side or until golden brown.
4. Push the sea bass fillets to one side of the skillet and add the remaining olive oil. Toss in the asparagus and cook until tender, about 4-5 minutes.
5. Reduce heat to low and add the herb-butter mixture to the skillet. Let it melt and baste the sea bass fillets with the melted herb butter.
6. Serve the herb-buttered sea bass fillets with asparagus. Drizzle any remaining herb butter from the skillet over the top.

Nutrition: Calories: 280; Fat: 15g; Carbs: 5g; Protein: 30g; Sugar: 1g; Fiber: 2g;

Equipment: Skillet; Small bowl; Spoon.

Carrot and Dill Hummus with Whole Grain Crackers

Prep time: 15 min   **Total time:** 15 min
Cook time: 0 min   **Servings:** 4

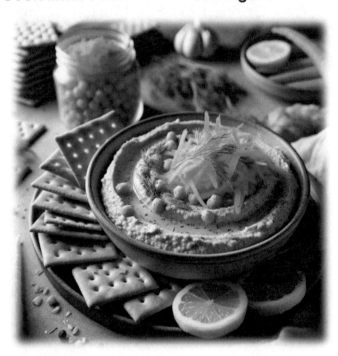

Ingredients:

- ✓ Chickpeas, cooked, 2 cups
- ✓ Carrot, grated, 1 cup
- ✓ Fresh dill, chopped, 2 tbsp
- ✓ Olive oil, 3 tbsp
- ✓ Lemon zest, 1 lemon
- ✓ Garlic cloves, 2 pcs
- ✓ Salt, 1 pinch
- ✓ Black pepper, 1 pinch
- ✓ Water, 1/4 cup
- ✓ Whole grain crackers (for serving)

Directions:

1. In a food processor, combine the chickpeas, grated carrot, chopped dill, lemon zest, and garlic cloves.
2. While the processor is running, slowly add in the olive oil and water. Blend until smooth.
3. Season with salt and black pepper, then pulse a few more times to mix.
4. Transfer to a serving bowl and serve with whole grain crackers.

Nutrition: Calories: 210; Fat: 9g; Carbs: 26g; Protein: 6g; Sugar: 4g; Fiber: 7g;

Equipment: Food processor; Serving bowl.

Mini Broccoli and Cheddar Quiches

Prep time: 20 min   **Total time:** 45 min
Cook time: 25 min   **Servings:** 6

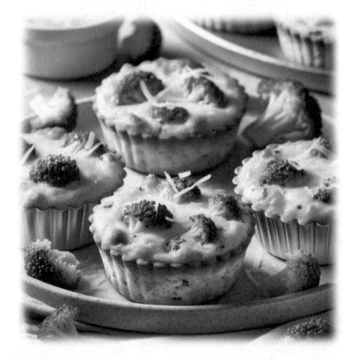

Ingredients:

- ✓ Broccoli, 1 cup (finely chopped)
- ✓ Eggs, 4 pcs
- ✓ Greek yogurt, 1/4 cup
- ✓ Grated Parmesan cheese, 1/2 cup
- ✓ Salt, 1 pinch
- ✓ Black pepper, 1 pinch
- ✓ Olive oil, 1 tbsp
- ✓ Water, 1 tbsp

Directions:

1. Preheat the oven to 375°F (190°C).
2. In a pan, heat the olive oil over medium heat. Add the finely chopped broccoli and sauté until slightly softened, about 3 minutes. Remove from heat and let it cool.
3. In a bowl, whisk together the eggs, Greek yogurt, grated Parmesan cheese, salt, black pepper, and water.
4. Fold in the sautéed broccoli.
5. Pour the mixture into mini quiche or muffin tins, filling each about 2/3 full.
6. Bake in the preheated oven for 20-25 minutes or until the quiches are set and the tops are lightly golden.
7. Allow to cool for a few minutes before serving.

Nutrition: Calories: 120; Fat: 7g; Carbs: 4g; Protein: 8g; Sugar: 1g; Fiber: 1g;

Equipment: Pan; Mixing bowl; Whisk; Mini quiche or muffin tins.

Baked Sweet Potato Fries with Avocado Dip

Prep time: 15 min   **Total time:** 45 min
Cook time: 30 min   **Servings:** 4

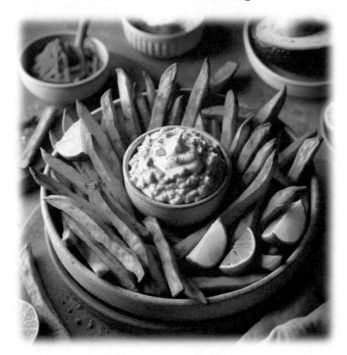

Ingredients:

✓ Sweet potatoes, 2 cups (peeled and thinly sliced)
✓ Olive oil, 2 tbsp
✓ Paprika, 1/2 tsp
✓ Salt, 1 pinch
✓ Black pepper, 1 pinch
✓ Avocado, 2 pcs
✓ Greek yogurt, 1/4 cup
✓ Lime zest, from 1 lime
✓ Garlic cloves, 2 pcs (minced)

Directions:

1. Preheat oven to 425°F (220°C).
2. In a large bowl, toss the sweet potato fries with olive oil, paprika, salt, and black pepper.
3. Spread the fries in a single layer on a baking sheet lined with parchment paper.
4. Bake in the preheated oven for 25-30 minutes or until crispy and golden brown, turning occasionally.
5. While the fries are baking, prepare the avocado dip. In a bowl, mash the avocados. Add Greek yogurt, lime zest, and minced garlic. Mix until smooth.
6. Serve the baked sweet potato fries with the avocado dip.

Nutrition: Calories: 260; Fat: 15g; Carbs: 30g; Protein: 4g; Sugar: 5g; Fiber: 7g;

Equipment: Oven; Large bowl; Baking sheet; Parchment paper; Mixing bowl.

Beetroot and Goat Cheese Tartlets

Prep time: 20 min   **Total time:** 45 min
Cook time: 25 min   **Servings:** 4

Ingredients:

✓ Beetroots, 1 cup (cooked and sliced)
✓ Olive oil, 1 tbsp
✓ Salt, 1 pinch
✓ Black pepper, 1 pinch

- ✓ Whole grain crackers, 8 (for serving)
- ✓ Feta cheese, crumbled, 1/2 cup
- ✓ Fresh thyme, chopped, 1 tbsp
- ✓ Honey, 1 tbsp
- ✓ Fresh basil leaves, 8 leaves (for garnish)

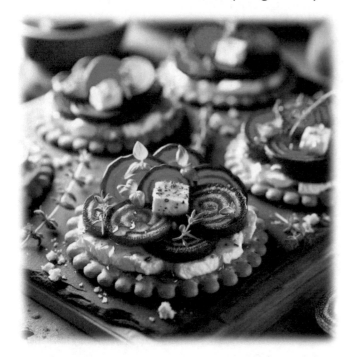

Spicy Roasted Chickpeas with Lime

Prep time: 10 min   **Total time:** 30 min
Cook time: 20 min   **Servings:** 4

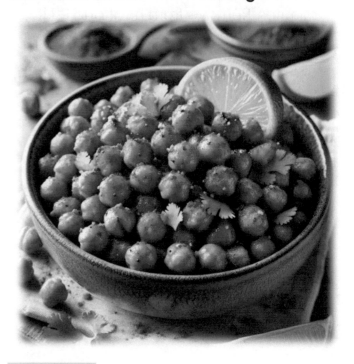

Directions:

1. Preheat oven to 375°F (190°C).
2. In a bowl, mix beetroots with olive oil, salt, and black pepper.
3. Arrange whole grain crackers on a baking tray.
4. Top each cracker with beetroot slices.
5. Sprinkle crumbled feta cheese over the beetroots.
6. Drizzle honey over each tartlet.
7. Bake in the preheated oven for about 10-12 minutes or until the cheese has slightly melted.
8. Remove from the oven and sprinkle fresh thyme on top.
9. Garnish with fresh basil leaves before serving.

Nutrition: Calories: 150; Fat: 8g; Carbs: 15g; Protein: 4g; Sugar: 7g; Fiber: 3g;

Equipment: Oven; Bowl; Baking tray.

Ingredients:

- ✓ Chickpeas, cooked, 2 cups
- ✓ Olive oil, 2 tbsp
- ✓ Paprika, 1 tsp
- ✓ Salt, 1 pinch
- ✓ Black pepper, 1 pinch
- ✓ Lime zest, 1 lime
- ✓ Fresh cilantro, chopped, 2 tbsp

Directions:

1. Preheat oven to 400°F (205°C).
2. In a bowl, combine chickpeas, olive oil, paprika, salt, and black pepper. Mix well to ensure chickpeas are evenly coated.
3. Spread chickpeas on a baking sheet in a single layer.
4. Roast in the preheated oven for 20 minutes or until crispy, stirring occasionally.
5. Once done, remove from the oven and transfer to a serving bowl.
6. Sprinkle with lime zest and chopped cilantro before serving.

Nutrition: Calories: 170; Fat: 9g; Carbs: 20g; Protein: 7g; Sugar: 3g; Fiber: 5g;

Equipment: Oven; Mixing bowl; Baking sheet.

Grilled Pineapple and Mint Skewers

Prep time: 10 min   **Total time:** 20 min
Cook time: 30 min   **Servings:** 4

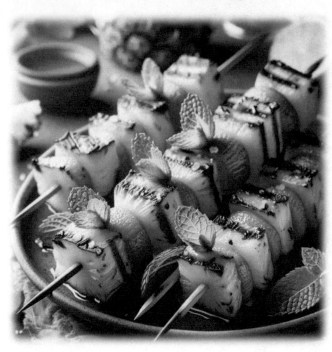

Ingredients:

✓ Fresh pineapple chunks, 2 cups
✓ Fresh mint leaves, 16 leaves
✓ Honey, 1 tbsp
✓ Lime zest, 1 lime
✓ Olive oil, 1 tbsp
✓ Salt, 1 pinch

Directions:

1. Preheat grill to medium-high heat.
2. In a bowl, mix together pineapple chunks, honey, lime zest, olive oil, and a pinch of salt. Toss to coat.
3. Thread pineapple chunks and fresh mint leaves alternately onto skewers.
4. Grill skewers for 4-5 minutes on each side or until pineapple is nicely charred.

5. Remove from the grill and serve immediately.

Nutrition: Calories: 90; Fat: 3g; Carbs: 16g; Protein: 1g; Sugar: 12g; Fiber: 1g;

Equipment: Grill; Mixing bowl; Skewers.

Stuffed Bell Peppers with Quinoa and Black Beans

Prep time: 15 min   **Total time:** 55 min
Cook time: 40 min   **Servings:** 4

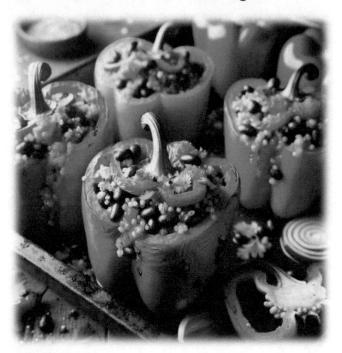

Ingredients:

✓ Red bell peppers, 4 pcs
✓ Quinoa, 1 cup
✓ Black beans, cooked, 2 cups
✓ Olive oil, 1 tbsp
✓ Red onion, thinly sliced, 1 cup
✓ Garlic cloves, 2 pcs
✓ Fresh cilantro, chopped, 2 tbsp
✓ Salt, 1 pinch
✓ Black pepper, 1 pinch
✓ Water, 2 cups

Directions:

1. Preheat the oven to 375°F (190°C).

2. Heat olive oil in a pan over medium heat. Add the red onion and garlic and sauté until translucent.
3. Add the quinoa, black beans, salt, and black pepper to the pan. Stir to combine.
4. Add water and bring the mixture to a boil. Reduce heat to low and simmer until quinoa is cooked and water is absorbed.
5. Remove from heat and stir in the fresh cilantro.
6. Carefully stuff each bell pepper with the quinoa and black bean mixture.
7. Place the stuffed peppers in a baking dish and bake for 20-25 minutes, or until the peppers are tender.
8. For decoration, you can reattach the previously cut stem to each bell pepper, adding a touch of color and enhancing the presentation of the dish.
9. Serve warm.

Nutrition: Calories: 310; Fat: 5g; Carbs: 55g; Protein: 12g; Sugar: 4g; Fiber: 9g;

Equipment: Oven; Pan; Baking dish.

DESSERT RECIPES

Berry Chia Seed Pudding

Prep time: 10 min   **Total time:** 10 min
Cook time: 0 min   **Servings:** 4

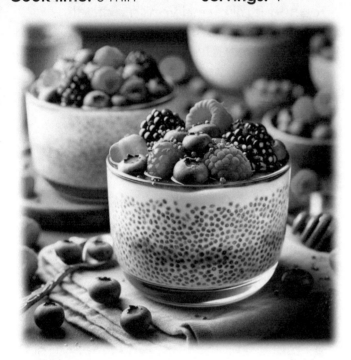

Ingredients:

✓ Chia seeds, 1/2 cup
✓ Greek yogurt, 2 cups
✓ Mixed fresh berries, 2 cups
✓ Honey, 2 tbsp
✓ Water, 1 cup
✓ Vanilla extract, 1 tsp
✓ Salt, a pinch

Directions:

1. In a mixing bowl, combine chia seeds, Greek yogurt, honey, vanilla extract, and a pinch of salt.
2. Gradually add water and stir until well combined.
3. Cover the bowl and refrigerate overnight, or for at least 4 hours.
4. Once the pudding has thickened, give it a good stir.

5. Divide the pudding into serving bowls.
6. Top each serving with a portion of mixed fresh berries.
7. Serve immediately or store in the fridge until ready to eat.

Nutrition: Calories: 220; Fat: 8g; Carbs: 30g; Protein: 10g; Sugar: 15g; Fiber: 10g;

Equipment: Mixing bowl; Spoon or spatula; Serving bowls.

Vanilla and Cinnamon Roasted Pears

Prep time: 10 min   **Total time:** 35 min
Cook time: 25 min   **Servings:** 4

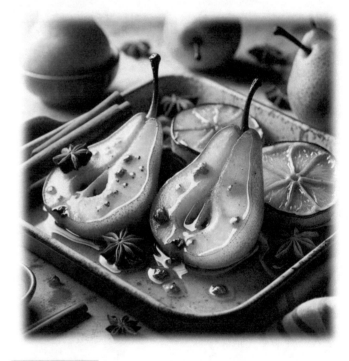

Ingredients:

✓ Fresh pears, halved and cored, 4 pcs
✓ Honey, 2 tbsp
✓ Cinnamon, 2 tsp
✓ Vanilla extract, 1 tsp
✓ Water, 1/2 cup
✓ Lemon zest, from 1 lemon

Directions:

1. Preheat the oven to 375°F (190°C).

2. In a small bowl, combine honey, cinnamon, vanilla extract, and lemon zest.
3. Arrange the pear halves, cut-side up, in a baking dish.
4. Drizzle the honey mixture over the pears.
5. Pour water into the base of the baking dish.
6. Roast in the oven for 20-25 minutes or until the pears are tender and the tops are caramelized.
7. Remove from the oven and let cool for a few minutes.
8. Serve the pears with a drizzle of the syrup from the baking dish.

Nutrition: Calories: 120; Fat: 0.2g; Carbs: 32g; Protein: 0.5g; Sugar: 26g; Fiber: 5g;

Equipment: Oven; Baking dish; Small bowl; Spoon or spatula.

Coconut Mango Mousse

Prep time: 15 min
Cook time: 0 min
Total time: 15 min
Servings: 4

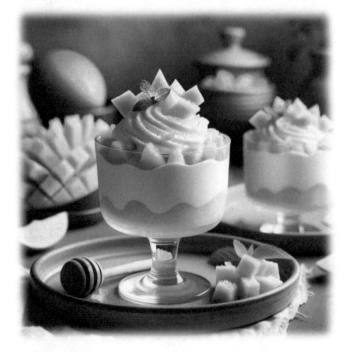

Ingredients:

✓ Fresh mango, 2 pcs
✓ Greek yogurt, 1 cup
✓ Honey, 2 tbsp
✓ Lime zest, from 1 lime
✓ Coconut milk (full fat), 1 cup
✓ Vanilla extract, 1 tsp

Directions:

1. Peel and chop the fresh mangoes, reserving a few cubes for garnish.
2. In a blender, combine the chopped mangoes, Greek yogurt, honey, lime zest, coconut milk, and vanilla extract.
3. Blend until smooth and creamy.
4. Pour the mousse into individual serving dishes or glasses.
5. Chill in the refrigerator for at least 1 hour before serving.
6. Garnish with reserved mango cubes before serving.

Nutrition: Calories: 250; Fat: 15g; Carbs: 28g; Protein: 5g; Sugar: 22g; Fiber: 3g;

Equipment: Blender; Peeler; Knife; Serving dishes or glasses.

Dark Chocolate Avocado Truffles

Prep time: 15 min
Cook time: 5 min
Total time: 45 min
Servings: 4

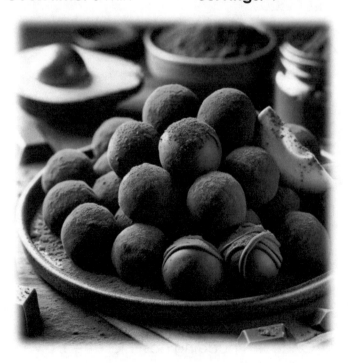

Ingredients:

- ✓ Dark chocolate (at least 70% cocoa), 6 oz
- ✓ Avocado, 1 pc (ripe)
- ✓ Vanilla extract, 1 tsp
- ✓ Cocoa powder, for rolling
- ✓ Salt, 1 pinch

Directions:

1. Melt the dark chocolate in a microwave or over a double boiler until smooth.
2. In a bowl, mash the ripe avocado until very smooth.
3. Mix the melted chocolate with the mashed avocado and add the vanilla extract and a pinch of salt. Stir until well combined.
4. Place the mixture in the refrigerator for about 30 minutes to firm up.
5. Once the mixture is firm, use a spoon to scoop out balls of the chocolate mixture and roll them into balls.
6. Roll the truffles in cocoa powder until fully coated.
7. Store in the refrigerator until ready to serve.

Nutrition: Calories: 90; Fat: 6g; Carbs: 7g; Protein: 1g; Sugar: 3g; Fiber: 2g;

Equipment: Bowl; Spoon; Microwave or double boiler.

Steamed Banana Bread with Walnuts

Prep time: 20 min
Cook time: 45 min
Total time: 65 min
Servings: 2

Ingredients:

- ✓ All-purpose flour, 1.5 cups
- ✓ Baking powder, 1 tsp
- ✓ Cinnamon, 1 tsp
- ✓ Salt, 1 pinch
- ✓ Eggs, 2 pcs
- ✓ Honey, 4 tbsp
- ✓ Bananas, ripe, 3 pcs (mashed)
- ✓ Toasted walnuts, 1 cup
- ✓ Vanilla extract, 1 tsp
- ✓ Water, for steaming

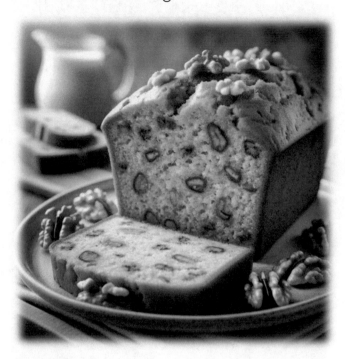

Directions:

1. In a large bowl, whisk together the all-purpose flour, baking powder, cinnamon, and salt.
2. In another bowl, beat the eggs, then add honey, mashed bananas, and vanilla extract. Mix until well combined.
3. Gradually add the wet ingredients to the dry ingredients, mixing just until incorporated.
4. Fold in the toasted walnuts.
5. Pour the batter into a greased steaming dish or loaf pan that fits inside your steamer.
6. Fill your steamer with water and bring to a boil.
7. Place the loaf pan inside the steamer, cover, and steam for about 45 minutes or until a toothpick inserted into the center comes out clean.
8. Let cool for a few minutes, then remove from the pan and slice to serve.

Nutrition: Calories: 240; Fat: 8g; Carbs: 37g; Protein: 5g; Sugar: 15g; Fiber: 3g;

Equipment: Large bowl; Steamer; Loaf pan or steaming dish.

Oat and Apple Crumble with Unsweetened Greek Yogurt

Prep time: 15 min
Cook time: 30 min

Total time: 45 min
Servings: 6

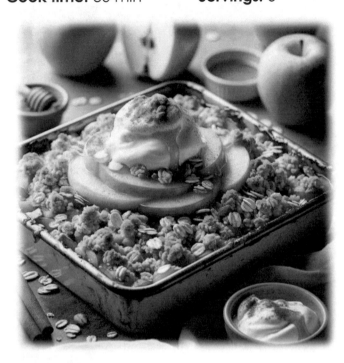

Ingredients:

- ✓ 3 Fresh apples, peeled and sliced
- ✓ 2 cups Rolled oats
- ✓ 1 tsp Cinnamon
- ✓ 1 tbsp Honey
- ✓ 2 tbsp Butter (unsalted), melted
- ✓ 2 cups Greek yogurt
- ✓ 1 pinch Salt
- ✓ 1 pinch Black pepper

Directions:

1. Preheat the oven to 350°F (175°C).
2. In a mixing bowl, combine rolled oats, cinnamon, honey, melted butter, salt, and black pepper. Mix until the oats are well-coated.
3. In a separate bowl, toss the apple slices with a bit of cinnamon.
4. Place the apple slices at the bottom of a baking dish.
5. Spread the oat mixture over the apples.
6. Bake in the oven for 30 minutes or until the top is golden brown and apples are tender.
7. Serve warm with a dollop of Greek yogurt on top.

Nutrition: Calories: 210; Fat: 6g; Carbs: 32g; Protein: 8g; Sugar: 10g; Fiber: 5g;

Equipment: Oven; Mixing bowl; Baking dish.

Blueberry and Lemon Zest Cheesecake Cups

Prep time: 20 min
Cook time: 180 min

Total time: 200 min
Servings: 6

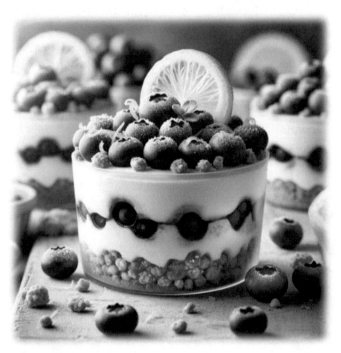

Ingredients:

- ✓ 1 cup Greek yogurt
- ✓ 1 cup Cottage cheese
- ✓ 1 Lemon zest
- ✓ 2 tbsp Honey
- ✓ 1 tsp Vanilla extract
- ✓ 1 cup Mixed fresh berries (mostly blueberries)
- ✓ 1 pinch Salt
- ✓ 6 Whole grain crackers, crushed

Directions:

1. In a blender, combine Greek yogurt, cottage cheese, lemon zest, honey, vanilla extract, and salt. Blend until smooth and creamy.
2. In serving cups or glasses, create a base layer using the crushed whole grain crackers.
3. Pour the cheesecake mixture over the cracker base.
4. Top with a generous amount of blueberries and other fresh berries.
5. Refrigerate for at least 3 hours or until set.
6. Serve chilled, garnished with a sprinkle of lemon zest.

Nutrition: Calories: 150; Fat: 3g; Carbs: 20g; Protein: 10g; Sugar: 8g; Fiber: 2g;

Equipment: Blender; Serving cups or glasses.

56-DAY MEAL PLAN

DAY	BREAKFAST	LUNCH	DINNER	SNACKS/ DESSERTS	CALORIES (kcal)
1	Honey Drizzle Oatmeal with Fresh Berries (11)	Crisp Cucumber Salad with Dill Vinaigrette (19)	Lemon-Pepper Baked Mackerel (47)	Carrot and Dill Hummus with Whole Grain Crackers (56)	840
2	Mango Greek Yogurt with Toasted Walnuts (11)	Fresh Herb and Cabbage Broth (28)	Lemon-Pepper Chicken Drumsticks (38)	Berry Chia Seed Pudding (61)	850
3	Raspberry and Oat Smoothie (17)	Tomato and Red Onion Salad with Cilantro (19)	Tilapia with Tomato-Basil Relish (47)	Mini Broccoli and Cheddar Quiches (56)	640
4	Fresh Fig and Cottage Cheese Toast (12)	Tofu and Mushroom Goulash in Tomato Sauce (33)	Grilled Turkey Patties with Lime and Cilantro (38)	Vanilla and Cinnamon Roasted Pears (61)	820
5	Broccoli and Mozzarella Omelette (12)	Apple and Celery Salad with Walnuts (20)	Garlic and Herb Crusted Whitefish (48)	Baked Sweet Potato Fries with Avocado Dip (57)	980
6	Apple and Cinnamon Whole Wheat Pita Pockets (13)	Tilapia Soup with Green Peas (28)	Spiced Beef Lettuce Wraps with Avocado (39)	Coconut Mango Mousse (62)	1010
7	Barley Breakfast Bowl with Pumpkin Seeds (13)	Mixed Bean Salad with Parsley and Feta (20)	Simple Shrimp and Broccoli Stir-Fry (48)	Beetroot and Goat Cheese Tartlets (57)	870
8	Golden Turmeric and Pineapple Smoothie (18)	Chickpea and Vegetable Goulash (33)	Herb-Infused Chicken Skewers with Cherry Tomatoes (39)	Dark Chocolate Avocado Truffles (62)	760
9	Baked Beans on Whole Grain Toast (14)	Mackerel and Cucumber Slaw with Dijon Dressing (21)	Honey-Mustard Glazed Pork Tenderloin (40)	Spicy Roasted Chickpeas with Lime (58)	1005
10	Zucchini and Cottage Cheese Pancakes (14)	Chicken and Barley Herb Soup (29)	Pan-Fried Catfish with Lemon Aioli (49)	Steamed Banana Bread with Walnuts (63)	1020
11	Baked Portobello Mushrooms with Eggs and Herbs (15)	Herring and Beetroot Salad with Fresh Dill (22)	Baked Turkey Sausage with Red Peppers and Onions (41)	Grilled Pineapple and Mint Skewers (59)	810
12	Spinach and Tomato Breakfast Wraps (16)	Sweet Potato and Black Bean Goulash (34)	Spiced Cod with Fresh Tomato Salsa (50)	Oat and Apple Crumble with Unsweetened Greek Yogurt (64)	995

DAY	BREAKFAST	LUNCH	DINNER	SNACKS/ DESSERTS	CALORIES (kcal)
13	Creamy Papaya and Spinach Smoothie (18)	Grilled Chicken and Peach Salad with Honey Vinaigrette (22)	Shrimp and Corn Quesadillas (50)	Stuffed Bell Peppers with Quinoa and Black Beans (59)	1140
14	Multi-seed Whole Grain Scones with Fresh Fruit (16)	Moroccan Spiced Lentil and Vegetable Soup (30)	Rosemary Beef Tips with Brussels Sprouts (41)	Blueberry and Lemon Zest Cheesecake Cups (64)	980
15	Honey Drizzle Oatmeal with Fresh Berries (11)	Spiced Turkey and Grape Salad with Feta Crumbles (23)	Baked Trout with Orange and Rosemary (51)	Carrot and Dill Hummus with Whole Grain Crackers (56)	970
16	Mango Greek Yogurt with Toasted Walnuts (11)	Chicken and Green Bean Goulash (35)	Ginger-Soy Glazed Haddock (52)	Berry Chia Seed Pudding (61)	1030
17	Raspberry and Oat Smoothie (17)	Broccoli and Cauliflower Salad with Lemon Zest (23)	Stuffed Chicken Thighs with Quinoa and Asparagus (42)	Mini Broccoli and Cheddar Quiches (56)	830
18	Fresh Fig and Cottage Cheese Toast (12)	Turkey Meatball and Spinach Soup (30)	Flounder Fillets with Cilantro and Lime (52)	Vanilla and Cinnamon Roasted Pears (61)	770
19	Broccoli and Mozzarella Omelette (12)	Charred Green Bean Salad with Garlic Aioli (24)	Lamb Meatballs with Mint and Lemon Zest (43)	Baked Sweet Potato Fries with Avocado Dip (57)	990
20	Apple and Cinnamon Whole Wheat Pita Pockets (13)	Shrimp and Broccoli Goulash in Lemon Herb Sauce (35)	Pomegranate-Glazed Chicken Wings (43)	Coconut Mango Mousse (62)	1000
21	Barley Breakfast Bowl with Pumpkin Seeds (13)	Smoked Salmon and Fennel Salad with Citrus Vinaigrette (25)	Shrimp Tacos with Cabbage Slaw (53)	Beetroot and Goat Cheese Tartlets (57)	990
22	Golden Turmeric and Pineapple Smoothie (18)	Rustic Mushroom and Thyme Soup (31)	Garlic Butter Roasted Cornish Hen (44)	Dark Chocolate Avocado Truffles (62)	920
23	Baked Beans on Whole Grain Toast (14)	Beef Strip and Roasted Brussels Sprouts Salad (25)	Baked Salmon Patties with Dill Sauce (53)	Spicy Roasted Chickpeas with Lime (58)	990
24	Zucchini and Cottage Cheese Pancakes (14)	Lentil and Swiss Chard Goulash (36)	Beef and Mushroom Stir-Fry with Broccoli (45)	Steamed Banana Bread with Walnuts (63)	1000
25	Baked Portobello Mushrooms with Eggs and Herbs (15)	Warm Lentil and Spinach Salad with Poached Eggs (26)	Grilled Red Snapper with Avocado and Mango Relish (54)	Grilled Pineapple and Mint Skewers (59)	790

DAY	BREAKFAST	LUNCH	DINNER	SNACKS/ DESSERTS	CALORIES (kcal)
26	Spinach and Tomato Breakfast Wraps (16)	Mediterranean Sea Bass Soup (32)	Cilantro-Lime Chicken with Avocado Salsa (45)	Oat and Apple Crumble with Unsweetened Greek Yogurt (64)	1045
27	Creamy Papaya and Spinach Smoothie (18)	Roasted Butternut Squash and Quinoa Salad with Cranberries (27)	Herb-Buttered Sea Bass with Asparagus (55)	Stuffed Bell Peppers with Quinoa and Black Beans (59)	1120
28	Multi-seed Whole Grain Scones with Fresh Fruit (16)	Cod and Asparagus Goulash with Parsley (37)	Smoked Paprika Pork Ribs with Roasted Vegetable Medley (46)	Blueberry and Lemon Zest Cheesecake Cups (64)	1140
29	Honey Drizzle Oatmeal with Fresh Berries (11)	Crisp Cucumber Salad with Dill Vinaigrette (19)	Lemon-Pepper Baked Mackerel (47)	Carrot and Dill Hummus with Whole Grain Crackers (56)	840
30	Mango Greek Yogurt with Toasted Walnuts (11)	Fresh Herb and Cabbage Broth (28)	Lemon-Pepper Chicken Drumsticks (38)	Berry Chia Seed Pudding (61)	850
31	Raspberry and Oat Smoothie (17)	Tomato and Red Onion Salad with Cilantro (19)	Tilapia with Tomato-Basil Relish (47)	Mini Broccoli and Cheddar Quiches (56)	640
32	Fresh Fig and Cottage Cheese Toast (12)	Tofu and Mushroom Goulash in Tomato Sauce (33)	Grilled Turkey Patties with Lime and Cilantro (38)	Vanilla and Cinnamon Roasted Pears (61)	820
33	Broccoli and Mozzarella Omelette (12)	Apple and Celery Salad with Walnuts (20)	Garlic and Herb Crusted Whitefish (48)	Baked Sweet Potato Fries with Avocado Dip (57)	980
34	Apple and Cinnamon Whole Wheat Pita Pockets (13)	Tilapia Soup with Green Peas (28)	Spiced Beef Lettuce Wraps with Avocado (39)	Coconut Mango Mousse (62)	1010
35	Barley Breakfast Bowl with Pumpkin Seeds (13)	Mixed Bean Salad with Parsley and Feta (20)	Simple Shrimp and Broccoli Stir-Fry (48)	Beetroot and Goat Cheese Tartlets (57)	870
36	Golden Turmeric and Pineapple Smoothie (18)	Chickpea and Vegetable Goulash (33)	Herb-Infused Chicken Skewers with Cherry Tomatoes (39)	Dark Chocolate Avocado Truffles (62)	760
37	Baked Beans on Whole Grain Toast (14)	Mackerel and Cucumber Slaw with Dijon Dressing (21)	Honey-Mustard Glazed Pork Tenderloin (40)	Spicy Roasted Chickpeas with Lime (58)	1005

DAY	BREAKFAST	LUNCH	DINNER	SNACKS/ DESSERTS	CALORIES (kcal)
38	Zucchini and Cottage Cheese Pancakes (14)	Chicken and Barley Herb Soup (29)	Pan-Fried Catfish with Lemon Aioli (49)	Steamed Banana Bread with Walnuts (63)	1020
39	Baked Portobello Mushrooms with Eggs and Herbs (15)	Herring and Beetroot Salad with Fresh Dill (22)	Baked Turkey Sausage with Red Peppers and Onions (41)	Grilled Pineapple and Mint Skewers (59)	810
40	Spinach and Tomato Breakfast Wraps (16)	Sweet Potato and Black Bean Goulash (34)	Spiced Cod with Fresh Tomato Salsa (50)	Oat and Apple Crumble with Unsweetened Greek Yogurt (64)	995
41	Creamy Papaya and Spinach Smoothie (18)	Grilled Chicken and Peach Salad with Honey Vinaigrette (22)	Shrimp and Corn Quesadillas (50)	Stuffed Bell Peppers with Quinoa and Black Beans (59)	1140
42	Multi-seed Whole Grain Scones with Fresh Fruit (16)	Moroccan Spiced Lentil and Vegetable Soup (30)	Rosemary Beef Tips with Brussels Sprouts (41)	Blueberry and Lemon Zest Cheesecake Cups (64)	980
43	Honey Drizzle Oatmeal with Fresh Berries (11)	Spiced Turkey and Grape Salad with Feta Crumbles (23)	Baked Trout with Orange and Rosemary (51)	Carrot and Dill Hummus with Whole Grain Crackers (56)	970
44	Mango Greek Yogurt with Toasted Walnuts (11)	Chicken and Green Bean Goulash (35)	Ginger-Soy Glazed Haddock (52)	Berry Chia Seed Pudding (61)	1030
45	Raspberry and Oat Smoothie (17)	Broccoli and Cauliflower Salad with Lemon Zest (23)	Stuffed Chicken Thighs with Quinoa and Asparagus (42)	Mini Broccoli and Cheddar Quiches (56)	830
46	Fresh Fig and Cottage Cheese Toast (12)	Turkey Meatball and Spinach Soup (30)	Flounder Fillets with Cilantro and Lime (52)	Vanilla and Cinnamon Roasted Pears (61)	770
47	Broccoli and Mozzarella Omelette (12)	Charred Green Bean Salad with Garlic Aioli (24)	Lamb Meatballs with Mint and Lemon Zest (43)	Baked Sweet Potato Fries with Avocado Dip (57)	990
48	Apple and Cinnamon Whole Wheat Pita Pockets (13)	Shrimp and Broccoli Goulash in Lemon Herb Sauce (35)	Pomegranate-Glazed Chicken Wings (43)	Coconut Mango Mousse (62)	1000
49	Barley Breakfast Bowl with Pumpkin Seeds (13)	Smoked Salmon and Fennel Salad with Citrus Vinaigrette (25)	Shrimp Tacos with Cabbage Slaw (53)	Beetroot and Goat Cheese Tartlets (57)	990
50	Golden Turmeric and Pineapple Smoothie (18)	Rustic Mushroom and Thyme Soup (31)	Garlic Butter Roasted Cornish Hen (44)	Dark Chocolate Avocado Truffles (62)	920

DAY	BREAKFAST	LUNCH	DINNER	SNACKS/ DESSERTS	CALORIES (kcal)
51	Baked Beans on Whole Grain Toast (14)	Beef Strip and Roasted Brussels Sprouts Salad (25)	Baked Salmon Patties with Dill Sauce (53)	Spicy Roasted Chickpeas with Lime (58)	990
52	Zucchini and Cottage Cheese Pancakes (14)	Lentil and Swiss Chard Goulash (36)	Beef and Mushroom Stir-Fry with Broccoli (45)	Steamed Banana Bread with Walnuts (63)	1000
53	Baked Portobello Mushrooms with Eggs and Herbs (15)	Warm Lentil and Spinach Salad with Poached Eggs (26)	Grilled Red Snapper with Avocado and Mango Relish (54)	Grilled Pineapple and Mint Skewers (59)	790
54	Spinach and Tomato Breakfast Wraps (16)	Mediterranean Sea Bass Soup (32)	Cilantro-Lime Chicken with Avocado Salsa (45)	Oat and Apple Crumble with Unsweetened Greek Yogurt (64)	1045
55	Creamy Papaya and Spinach Smoothie (18)	Roasted Butternut Squash and Quinoa Salad with Cranberries (27)	Herb-Buttered Sea Bass with Asparagus (55)	Stuffed Bell Peppers with Quinoa and Black Beans (59)	1120
56	Multi-seed Whole Grain Scones with Fresh Fruit (16)	Cod and Asparagus Goulash with Parsley (37)	Smoked Paprika Pork Ribs with Roasted Vegetable Medley (46)	Blueberry and Lemon Zest Cheesecake Cups (64)	1140

COOKING CONVERSION CHART

Volume Equivalents (Dry)

US Standard	Metric (approximate)
1/8 teaspoon	0.5 mL
1/4 teaspoon	1 mL
1/2 teaspoon	2 mL
3/4 teaspoon	4 mL
1 teaspoon	5 mL
1 tablespoon	15 mL
1/4 cup	59 mL
1/3 cup	79 mL
1/2 cup	118 mL
2/3 cup	156 mL
3/4 cup	177 mL
1 cup	235 mL
2 cups or 1 pint	475 mL
3 cups	700 mL
4 cups or 1 quart	1 L

Volume Equivalents (Liquid)

US Standard	US Standard (ounces)	Metric (approximate)
2 tablespoons	1 fl. oz.	30 mL
1/4 cup	2 fl. oz.	60 mL
1/2 cup	4 fl. oz.	120 mL
1 cup	8 fl. oz.	240 mL
1 1/2 cup	12 fl. oz.	355 mL
2 cups or 1 pint	16 fl. oz.	475 mL
4 cups or 1 quart	32 fl. oz.	1 L
1 gallon	128 fl. oz.	4 L

Oven Temperatures

Fahrenheit (F)	Celsius (C) (approximate)
250	120
300	150
325	165
350	180
375	190
400	200
425	220
450	230

Weight Equivalents

US Standard	Metric (approximate)
1/2 ounce	15 g
1 ounce	30 g
2 ounces	60 g
4 ounces	115 g
8 ounces	225 g
12 ounces	340 g
16 ounces or 1 pound	455 g

Ingredient	Quantity	Unit
Avocado	1 1/2	pcs
Barley	1/2	cup
Beef strip steak	8	oz
Beetroots	1/2	cups
Black pepper	3/4	tsp
Broccoli	2 1/2	cup
Canned baked beans	1	cups
Carrot, grated	1/2	cups
Celery, thinly sliced	1	cup
Cherry tomatoes	3 1/2	cups
Chia seeds	1/4	cup
Chicken drumsticks	4	pcs
Chickpeas, cooked	1	cups
Chopped fresh parsley	2	tbsp
Chopped nuts	1/2	cup
Cinnamon	1 1/2	tsp
Coconut milk (full fat)	1/2	cup
Cod fillets	2	oz
Cottage cheese	1	cup
Cucumbers, thinly sliced	1	cups
Eggs	6	pcs
Feta cheese, crumbled	3/4	cup
Firm tofu, cubed	7	oz
Fresh apples	2	pcs
Fresh basil leaves	9	leaves
Fresh cilantro, chopped	5	tbsp
Fresh dill, chopped	4	tbsp
Fresh figs	4	pcs
Fresh mackerel fillets	2	pcs
Fresh mango	2	pc
Fresh pears, halved and cored	2	pcs
Fresh raspberries	1	cup
Fresh rosemary, finely chopped	1	tbsp
Fresh spinach	1	cups
Fresh thyme (chopped)	2	tbsp
Garlic cloves	16	pcs
Grated Parmesan cheese	1/6	cups
Greek yogurt	6	cups
Green cabbage, shredded	1	cups
Green peas	1	cups
Ground turkey	1/2	lb
Honey	1	cup

Lemon zest	5	lemon
Lime zest	2 1/2	limes
Mint leaves	9	leaves
Mixed fresh berries	2	cup
Mozzarella cheese	1/2	cup
Olive oil	1	cup
Paprika	3/4	tsp
Portobello mushrooms	2	large caps
Pumpkin seeds	1/4	cup
Red bell peppers, sliced	1/2	cup
Red onion, thinly sliced	1 1/2	cup
Rolled oats	1 1/2	cup
Salt	3/4	tsp
Shrimp, peeled and deveined	1/2	lb
Soy sauce (low sodium)	1	tbsp
Sweet potatoes	1	cups
Tilapia fillets	14	oz
Toasted walnuts	3/4	cup
Vanilla extract	1 1/2	tsp
Water	11	cups
White wine vinegar	2	tbsp
Whole grain bread	3	slices
Whole grain crackers	4	for serving
Whole wheat pita pockets	2	pcs

Ingredient	Quantity	Unit
All-purpose flour	1 1/2	cup
Avocado	1/2	pcs
Baking powder	1 1/2	tsp
Bananas, ripe	1 1/2	pcs
Barley	1/2	cups
Beef strip steak, cubed	8	oz
Beetroots, cooked and diced	1	cups
Black beans, cooked	2	cups
Black pepper	1	tsp
Brussels sprouts, halved	1	cups
Butter (unsalted)	2/3	tbsp
Butternut squash, peeled, seeded and diced	2/3	cups
Canned baked beans	1	cup
Carrot, grated	1 1/4	cup
Catfish fillets	12	oz
Celery, thinly sliced	2	cup

Cherry tomatoes	4	cup
Chicken drumsticks	4	pcs
Chickpeas, cooked	2	cups
Chopped fresh parsley	3 3/4	tbsp
Chopped nuts	1/8	cup
Cinnamon	1 1/4	tsp
Cocoa powder		For rolling
Cod fillets	12	oz
Cottage cheese	6/7	cup
Cucumbers, thinly sliced	1	cups
Dark chocolate (at least 70% cocoa)	3	oz
Dijon mustard	2	tsp
Dried green lentils	1/3	cup
Eggs	7	pcs
Fresh apples	1	pcs
Fresh cilantro, chopped	7	tbsp
Fresh dill, chopped	2 1/2	tbsp
Fresh herring fillets, marinated and chopped	2	pcs
Fresh mackerel fillets, grilled and flaked	2	pcs
Fresh mint leaves	8	leaves
Fresh peaches, halved and pitted	2	pcs
Fresh pineapple chunks	2	cup
Fresh rosemary, finely chopped	1	tbsp
Fresh spinach	5	cups
Fresh thyme (chopped)	2	tbsp
Garlic cloves	14	pcs
Grated Parmesan cheese	2/5	cup
Greek yogurt	4	cup
Green peas	1/2	cup
Grilled chicken breasts, sliced	4	pcs
Honey	3/4	cup
Ice cubes	1	cup
Lemon zest	2	lemon
Lime zest	2	lime
Mixed fresh berries	3/5	cup
Mozzarella cheese	1	cups
Olive oil	1 1/4	cups
Papaya, peeled and deseeded	1	cup
Paprika	2 1/2	tsp
Pork tenderloin	1/2	lb
Portobello mushrooms	2	large caps
Pumpkin seeds	0	cup
Quinoa	1/2	cup

Red bell peppers, sliced	3	cups
Red onion, thinly sliced	4	cup
Rolled oats	1	cup
Salt	3/4	tsp
Shrimp, peeled and deveined	1/2	lb
Sweet potatoes, peeled and diced	1 1/2	cups
Toasted walnuts	1/2	cups
Turkey sausage	1/2	lb
Turmeric powder	1 1/2	tsp
Vanilla extract	1 1/2	tsp
Water	12	cup
White wine vinegar	1 1/2	tbsp
Whole grain bread	2	slices
Whole grain crackers	2	pcs
Whole wheat pita pockets	4	pcs
Zucchini, grated	2 1/4	cups

SHOPPING LISTS WEEKS 3 AND 7 *

Ingredient	Quantity	Unit
Avocado	1	pcs
Barley	1/2	cup
Beetroots	1/2	cups
Black pepper	1/2	tsp
Broccoli	4 1/2	cup
Carrot, grated	6/7	cup
Cauliflower	2	cups
Celery, thinly sliced	1/3	cup
Cherry tomatoes	3/4	cups
Chia seeds	1/4	cup
Chicken drumsticks, boneless and skinless	10	pcs
Chickpeas, cooked	1	cups
Chopped nuts	1/2	cup
Cinnamon	1 3/4	tsp
Coconut milk (full fat)	1/2	cup
Cottage cheese	1	cup
Dijon mustard	1	tsp
Eggs	7	pcs
Fennel bulb	1/2	pcs
Feta cheese, crumbled	3/4	cup
Flounder fillets	12	oz
Fresh apples	1	pcs
Fresh asparagus, trimmed and chopped	1/2	cup

Ingredient		
Fresh basil leaves	4	leaves
Fresh cilantro, chopped	2 1/2	tbsp
Fresh dill, chopped	4 1/4	tbsp
Fresh figs	4	pcs
Fresh ginger, grated	1/2	tbsp
Fresh mango	2	pc
Fresh mint leaves, finely chopped	18	leaves
Fresh pears, halved and cored	2	pcs
Fresh raspberries	1	cup
Fresh rosemary, finely chopped	1/2	tbsp
Fresh spinach	5	cups
Fresh thyme, chopped	2	tbsp
Fresh trout fillets	2	oz each
Garlic cloves	13	pcs
Grated Parmesan cheese	1/6	cups
Greek yogurt	6 1/2	cups
Green beans	3	cups
Green cabbage	1	cups
Grilled chicken breasts, sliced	2	pcs
Ground lamb	1/2	lb
Ground turkey	6/7	lb
Haddock fillets	12	oz
Honey	1 1/8	cups
Lemon zest	4	lemon
Lime zest	2	lime
Mint leaves	9	leaves
Mixed fresh berries	2	cup
Mozzarella cheese	1/2	cup
Olive oil	1 1/8	cups
Orange, zested and juiced	1/2	pc
Paprika	3/4	tsp
Pomegranate juice	1/2	cup
Pumpkin seeds	1/4	cup
Quinoa	1/2	cup
Red grapes, halved	1	cups
Red onion, thinly sliced	2 1/4	cup
Rolled oats	1 1/2	cup
Salt	3/4	tsp
Shrimp, peeled and deveined	1	lb
Smoked salmon	4	oz
Soy sauce (low sodium)	2	tbsp
Sweet potatoes	1	cups

Ingredient		
Toasted walnuts	1/4	cup
Turmeric powder	1/4	tsp
Vanilla extract	1 1/2	tsp
Water	10 1/2	cups
White wine vinegar	2	tbsp
Whole grain bread	2	slices
Whole grain crackers	4	for serving
Whole wheat pita pockets	4	pcs

SHOPPING LISTS WEEKS 4 AND 8 *

Ingredient	Quantity	Unit
All-purpose flour	1 1/4	cup
Avocado	3	pcs
Baking powder	1 1/2	tsp
Bananas, ripe	1 1/2	pcs
Beef strip steak	16	oz
Black beans, cooked	1	cups
Black pepper	13	pinch
Broccoli	2	cups
Brussels sprouts	1	cups
Butter (unsalted)	1 3/4	tbsp
Butternut squash, peeled, seeded and diced	1	cups
Canned baked beans	1	cup
Carrot, grated	2	cup
Cauliflower	1	cups
Celery, thinly sliced	1	cup
Cherry tomatoes	2	cup
Chickpeas, cooked	1	cups
Chopped fresh parsley	5	tbsp
Chopped nuts	1/8	cup
Cinnamon	1	tsp
Cocoa powder	0	For rolling
Cod fillets	12	oz
Cornish hens	2	pcs
Cottage cheese	1	cup
Dark chocolate (at least 70% cocoa)	3	oz
Dijon mustard	2	tsp
Dried cranberries	1/4	cup
Dried green lentils	1	cup
Eggs	10	pcs
Feta cheese, crumbled	1/4	cup

Fresh apples	1 1/2	pcs
Fresh asparagus	2	cups
Fresh cilantro, chopped	4 1/2	tbsp
Fresh dill, chopped	2	tbsp
Fresh mango	1	pcs
Fresh mint leaves	8	leaves
Fresh pineapple chunks	2	cup
Fresh rosemary, finely chopped	3	tbsp
Fresh spinach	6	cups
Fresh thyme (chopped)	3 1/2	tbsp
Garlic cloves	19	pcs
Grated Parmesan cheese	2/5	cup
Greek yogurt	3 1/2	cup
Grilled chicken breasts	2	pcs
Honey	10	tbsp
Ice cubes	1	cup
Lemon zest	4	lemon
Lime zest	2	lime
Mixed fresh berries	3/5	cup
Olive oil	24	tbsp
Papaya, peeled and deseeded	1	cup
Paprika	2 1/2	tsp
Pork ribs	1	lb
Portobello mushrooms	6	large caps
Pumpkin seeds	0	cup
Quinoa	1	cup
Red bell peppers, sliced	3	cup
Red onion, thinly sliced	3 1/2	cup
Red snapper fillets	12	oz
Rolled oats	1	cup
Salt	14	pinch
Sea bass fillets	24	oz
Smoked salmon	12	oz
Soy sauce (low sodium)	1	tbsp
Swiss chard	2	cups
Toasted walnuts	1/2	cups
Turmeric powder	1	tsp
Vanilla extract	1 1/2	tsp
Water	13 1/2	cup
White wine vinegar	2	tbsp
Whole grain bread	3	slices
Whole grain crackers	2	pcs
Whole wheat pita pockets	2	pcs
Zucchini, grated	1	cups

* Understanding Your Mediterranean Diet Weekly Shopping List

- **Servings:** The quantities listed are calculated for two servings. So, if you're cooking for one, simply halve the quantities. For more servings, multiply accordingly.

- **Optional Items:** Ingredients marked as "optional," "to taste," or "as desired" in recipes may not be included in this list. Feel free to add them as you wish.

- **Rounded Measurements:** The quantities may be rounded up or down to match standard units. For example, if a recipe calls for a third of a cup, it's rounded to the nearest standard measurement for your convenience.

- **Substitutions:** If you have dietary restrictions or just don't like certain items, feel free to swap them out. For instance, almond milk can often be exchanged for dairy milk.

- **Storage:** Be aware of perishable items and consider storage. For example, fresh herbs can spoil quickly, so you may want to opt for dried versions if you don't plan to use them right away.

- **Local Availability:** Some Mediterranean ingredients might not be as readily available in all U.S. locations. Look for substitutes that maintain the spirit of the Mediterranean diet—think fresh, unprocessed, and colorful.

Keep this list handy when you go shopping, and feel free to tweak it to match your personal preferences and needs. Happy cooking!

INDEX

Conclusion

As we reach the end of this culinary guide, I'd like to offer my heartfelt gratitude for allowing me into your kitchen and daily life. The DASH diet, while being rooted in science and health principles, is so much more than just a diet. It's a lifestyle, a commitment to cherishing our health, and a journey to rediscovering the joy in wholesome, nourishing meals.

Remember, every step you take towards a healthier lifestyle is a victory, no matter how small. Whether you've decided to plunge headfirst into the DASH diet or are taking baby steps by incorporating a few recipes here and there, you are making a positive change.

This book was crafted with love, care, and a deep desire to provide not only delicious but also health-promoting meals. I hope that as you tried each recipe, you not only delighted in their flavors but also felt the passion and thoughtfulness with which they were curated.

In times when you might find it challenging, revisit these pages, find inspiration in the vibrant photographs, and remember why you started this journey. Health, vitality, and joy in the simple act of eating are gifts that keep on giving.

Thank you for being a part of this adventure with me. May your days be filled with delightful meals, joyous moments, and the deep satisfaction that comes with taking care of oneself.

To good health and delicious memories,

Ava Fit

Copyright © 2024 by Ava Fit

All rights reserved. No part of this book may be reproduced, distributed, or transmitted in any form or by any means, including photocopying, recording, or other electronic or mechanical methods, without the prior written permission of the publisher, except in the case of brief quotations embodied in critical reviews and certain other noncommercial uses permitted by copyright law.

Legal Notice. The information contained in this book is intended for educational and informational purposes only and is not a substitute for professional medical advice or treatment. Consult with a qualified healthcare professional before making any changes to your diet or lifestyle. The author and publisher expressly disclaim responsibility for any adverse effects that may result from the use or application of the information contained in this book.

Disclaimer. While every effort has been made to ensure the accuracy and reliability of the information contained in this book, neither the author nor the publisher can assume responsibility for errors, inaccuracies, or omissions. The reader is advised to consult with healthcare providers for specific health-related issues and should exercise caution when preparing recipes, particularly for allergies and dietary restrictions.

FREE BONUS

Dear Friend,

Thank you for choosing "The Dash Diet Cookbook for Beginners" as your guide on this inspiring journey to improved health and wellness. By adopting the DASH diet, you're not just changing your eating habits; you're embracing a lifestyle proven to support heart health and overall well-being. This diet, rich in diverse, nutritious foods, aligns perfectly with a heart-healthy lifestyle, supported by extensive scientific research.

To claim your **80+ BONUS MEDITERRANEAN DIET PDF RECIPES**, please send an email to **the.nutrabook@gmail.com** with your Amazon order number. We will promptly send you the bonus recipes. We are dedicated to enhancing your culinary journey and health with each book we publish. Your satisfaction motivates us to continually refine and improve our offerings. We highly value your feedback, suggestions, and constructive criticism, so please feel free to share your thoughts with us at the same email address. Your input is invaluable to us.

As you delve into the world of health-conscious eating, remember that "The Dash Diet Cookbook for Beginners" is just one part of a wider array of resources we offer.

We have a small favor to ask. As a small, independent publisher, every review is incredibly important to us. Your insights not only inspire us to keep enhancing our work but also help others make informed decisions. If you find value and insight in both this book and the bonus recipes, could you please take a moment to share your experience by leaving a review on Amazon? Your thoughts can greatly assist others who are on the same path to healthier living.

Your opinion is a guiding light for others on their health journey, and we are deeply grateful for your help in lighting the way.

Thank you for letting us be a part of your culinary and health journey. We wish you continued health and enjoyment as you explore the benefits of the DASH diet lifestyle.

With heartfelt gratitude,

Nutra Book Team

Made in United States
Troutdale, OR
09/15/2024

22850046R00044